MEASUREMENT IN ULTRASOUND

MEASUREMENT IN ULTRASOUND

A practical handbook

Paul S. Sidhu BSc MB BS MRCP FRCR DTM&H
Consultant Radiologist
Department of Radiology
King's College Hospital
London, UK

Wui K. Chong MB BS MRCP FRCR
Assistant Professor
University of North Carolina Hospital
Department of Radiology
Chapel Hill
North Carolina, USA

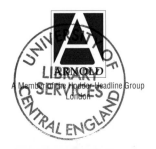

ARNOLD
A Member of the Hodder Headline Group
London

First published in Great Britain in 2004 by
Arnold, a member of the Hodder Headline Group,
338 Euston Road, London NW1 3BH

http://www.arnoldpublishers.com

Distributed in the United States of America by
Oxford University Press Inc.,
198 Madison Avenue, New York, NY10016
Oxford is a registered trademark of Oxford University Press

Whilst the advice and information in this book are believed to be true and
accurate at the date of going to press, neither the authors nor the publisher
can accept any legal responsibility or liability for any errors or omissions
that may be made. In particular (but without limiting the generality of the
preceding disclaimer) every effort has been made to check drug dosages;
however, it is still possible that errors have been missed. Furthermore,
dosage schedules are constantly being revised and new side-effects
recognized. For these reasons the reader is strongly urged to consult the
drug companies' printed instructions before administering any of the drugs
recommended in this book.

British Library Cataloguing in Publication Data
A catalogue record for this book is available from the British Library

Library of Congress Cataloging-in-Publication Data
A catalog record for this book is available from the Library of Congress

ISBN 0 340 76258 6

1 2 3 4 5 6 7 8 9 10

Commissioning Editor: Joanna Koster
Project Editor: Wendy Rooke
Production Controller: Debbie Smith
Cover Designer: Sarah Rees

Typeset in 9 on 11pt Sabon by Phoenix Photosetting, Chatham, Kent
Printed and bound in Italy

What do you think about this book? Or any other Arnold title?
Please send your comments to feedback.arnold@hodder.co.uk

CONTENTS

List of contributors   xi
Foreword by David O. Cosgrove   xiii
Foreword by Carol A. Mittelstaedt   xv
Preface   xvii
Acknowledgements   xviii

1 ABDOMEN (LIVER, GALLBLADDER AND SPLEEN)   1
Keshthra Satchithananda, Zelena A. Aziz, Maria E.K. Sellars and
Paul S. Sidhu

Liver (adult)   2
Liver (pediatric)   4
Gallbladder (adult)   6
Gallbladder (pediatric)   8
Gallbladder (neonatal)   10
Gallbladder wall   12
Common bile duct (adult)   14
Common bile duct (pediatric)   18
Hepatic duct (adult)   20
Spleen (adult and pediatric)   22
Diaphragmatic motion   26

2 ABDOMEN (VASCULAR)   29
Zelena A. Aziz, Keshthra Satchithananda and Paul S. Sidhu

Renal artery   30
Evaluation of acute renal obstruction with intrarenal Doppler   34
Portal vein   36
Hepatic veins   38
Hepatic artery   40
Celiac and superior mesenteric arteries   42
Doppler ultrasound measurement of postprandial intestinal
    blood flow   46
Inferior mesenteric artery   48

3 RETROPERITONEUM   51
Zelena A. Aziz, Keshthra Satchithananda, Maria E.K. Sellars and
Paul S. Sidhu

Kidneys (adult)   52
Kidney size (pediatric)   56

Kidney size (infant and neonatal)   60
Renal pelvic diameter (neonatal and fetal)   64
Adrenal glands (adult)   66
Adrenal glands (infant)   67
Adrenal glands (neonatal)   68
Pancreas (adult)   70
Pancreatic duct (adult)   72
Pancreas (pediatric)   74
Psoas muscle   76
Retroperitoneal lymph nodes   78

4   ORGAN TRANSPLANTATION   81

Keshthra Satchithananda, Zelena A. Aziz and Paul S. Sidhu

Kidney transplantation   82
Renal artery stenosis in transplantation   86
Liver transplantation   88
Pancreas transplantation   92

5   PELVIS   95
Bladder

Keshthra Satchithananda, Zelena A. Aziz and Paul S. Sidhu

Bladder volume and residual volume   96
Bladder wall   100
Ureterovesical jets (pediatric and infant)   102

Male genital tract   104

Zelena A. Aziz, Keshthra Satchithananda and Paul S. Sidhu

Testes   104
Epididymis   108
Prostate – transrectal sonography   110
Seminal vesicles – transrectal sonography   112
Penis   114

Female urogenital tract   118

Kelley Z. Allison and Wui K. Chong

Ovary – transvaginal sonography   118
Ovarian follicles – transvaginal sonography   120
Cervix – transvaginal sonography   122
Uterus – transvaginal sonography   124

Endometrial stripe – transvaginal sonography   126
Urethra   128
Length of the cervix and cervical canal in pregnancy   130

6   SUPERFICIAL STRUCTURES   133
Keshthra Satchithananda, Zelena A. Aziz and Paul S. Sidhu

Parathyroid glands   134
Submandibular salivary glands   136
Parotid salivary glands   138
Thyroid gland   140
Lymph nodes in the neck   144
Orbits – extraocular muscles   148
Orbits – optic nerve   150

7   NEONATAL BRAIN   153
Maria E.K. Sellars, Wui K. Chong and Paul S. Sidhu

Ventricular size   154
Doppler studies of intercranial blood flow   158

8   GASTROINTESTINAL TRACT   161
Zelena A. Aziz, Keshthra Satchithananda, Maria E.K. Sellars and
Paul S. Sidhu

Pyloric stenosis   162
Appendix   164
Upper gastrointestinal tract wall – endoscopic ultrasound   166
Bowel wall – transabdominal ultrasound   168
Anal endosonography   170

9   MUSCULOSKELETAL SYSTEM   173
Keshthra Satchithananda and David Elias

General considerations   174

Upper limb – shoulder   176
Long head of biceps   176
Subscapularis tendon   178
Supraspinatus tendon   180
Infraspinatus tendon   182

Upper limb – elbow   184
Anterior joint space   184
Olecranon fossa   186

Lateral elbow 188
Medial elbow 190

Upper limb – wrist **192**
Dorsal tendons 192
Carpal tunnel 194

Lower limb – hips **196**
Hip effusion 196
Developmental dysplasia of the hip 198

Lower limb – knee **200**

Lower limb – ankle **202**
Anterior, medial, lateral tendons 202
Achilles tendon 204

Lower limb – foot **206**
Plantar fascia 206
Interdigital web spaces 208

10 PERIPHERAL VASCULAR SYSTEM (ARTERIAL) **211**
Zelena A. Aziz and Paul S. Sidhu

Upper limbs – peripheral arteries 212
Abdominal aorta and common iliac arteries 214
Lower limbs – peripheral arteries 218
Lower limbs – peripheral arteries for stenosis 220
Extracranial arteries 222
Extracranial arteries – measurement of internal carotid
    artery stenosis 226
Transcranial Doppler ultrasound 230

11 PERIPHERAL VASCULAR SYSTEM (VENOUS) **235**
Paul S. Sidhu

Inferior vena cava 236
Neck veins 238
Leg veins 240

12 OBSTETRICS **243**
Wui K. Chong, Anthony E. Swartz and Janice Newsome

Comparison of serum β-hCG levels and ultrasound
    landmarks to gestational age on transvaginal sonography
    (first trimester) 244

Gestational sac (first trimester)   246
Fetal heartbeat (first trimester)   250
Crown–rump length   252
Nuchal fold thickness   254
Nuchal translucency thickness   256
Biparietal diameter   258
Head circumference   262
Abdominal circumference   266
Multiple fetal parameters in the assessment of gestational age   270
Ratio of head to abdomen circumference   274
Estimated fetal weight based on biparietal diameter and
    abdominal circumference   276
Fetal femur length   286
Fetal humerus length   290
Systolic/diastolic ratio in the umbilical artery   294
Cerebral ventricles – lateral ventricle transverse atrial
    measurement   298
Cisterna magna   300
Thoracic circumference   302
Renal pelvis diameter   304
Mean renal lengths for gestational ages   306
Outer orbital diameter   308
Fetal stomach diameter   312
Fetal small bowel   314
Fetal colon   316
Predicted fetal weight percentiles throughout pregnancy   318
Amniotic fluid   320

Index   323

CONTRIBUTORS

Kelley Z. Allison MD
Diagnostic Radiology,
Medical College of Virginia Hospitals,
Virginia Commonwealth University,
Virginia, USA

Zelena A. Aziz BSc MB BS MRCP FRCR
Department of Radiology,
King's College Hospital,
London, UK

Wui K. Chong MB BS MRCP FRCR
University of North Carolina Hospital,
Department of Radiology,
Chapel Hill, North Carolina, USA

David Elias MB BS MRCP FRCR
Department of Radiology,
King's College Hospital,
London, UK

Janice Newsome MD
Potomac Radiology, Alexandria,
Virginia, USA

Keshthra Satchithananda BDS FDSRCS MB BS FRCS FRCR
Department of Radiology,
King's College Hospital,
London, UK

Maria E.K. Sellars MBChB FRCR
Department of Radiology,
King's College Hospital,
London, UK

Paul S. Sidhu BSc MB BS MRCP FRCR DTM&H
Department of Radiology,
King's College Hospital,
London, UK

Anthony E. Swartz RT(R) RDMS
Department of Obstetrics and Gynecology,
University of North Carolina Hospital,
Chapel Hill, North Carolina, USA

FOREWORD BY DAVID O. COSGROVE

Measurements are needed for all imaging techniques to demonstrate that structures of interest are normal or abnormal and to document the degree of any abnormality. All too often, however, the normal values are buried in reference textbooks and may be awkward to find when they are needed during a busy scanning list. This pocket book corrects this defect by providing, in compact form, a comprehensive set of normal ultrasound measurements both for paediatrics and adults. The clearly ordered sections should make it simple and quick to locate the relevant information required and, for those who need to know more, selective references and suggestions for further reading are provided. Much of the normal value data is presented as convenient tables, particularly in the paediatrics sections.

The authors are well known researchers in imaging and particularly in ultrasound, Dr Sidhu in the UK and Dr Chong in the USA.

This book is highly commended to all working in the field of ultrasound: it will provide a valuable companion to routine clinical practice.

David O. Cosgrove
Professor of Clinical Ultrasound
Imaging Sciences Department
Faculty of Medicine
Imperial College
Hammersmith Hospital
London
UK

FOREWORD BY CAROL A. MITTELSTAEDT

The technology and applications of diagnostic ultrasound have shown remarkable growth since ultrasound was first used as a diagnostic imaging modality. Along with this expansion have been studies identifying appropriate ultrasound techniques and measurements. Though there have been numerous articles and books in the field of ultrasound, the readers of these must ferret out the measurements from the various publications. Until now there has been no 'quick' ultrasound measurement guide.

Measurement in Ultrasound is an excellent resource for those performing and interpreting ultrasound of all types. Not only are various measurements listed for a number of organs and structures for both pediatric and adult patients, but the ultrasound techniques employed to obtain these measurements are also described. Doppler parameters for a number of organs, such as transplants and various vessels, are defined along with the technique to obtain these.

This publication encompasses the abdomen (parenchymal organs and vessels), retroperitoneum, organ transplantation, male and female genital tracts, superficial structures (such as thyroid, lymph nodes, salivary glands), neonatal brain, gastrointestinal tract, musculoskeletal system, peripheral vascular system (both arterial and venous), and obstetrics. Each specific section describes the preparation, position, transducer, method, appearance, and measurement variables involved. With respect to obstetrics, this measurement handbook is a quick reference listing such variables as gestational sac size, relationship to heartbeat, gestational age, and more. Multiple measurements and Doppler parameters are provided for the obstetric patient.

My congratulations go to the authors of *Measurement in Ultrasound*, and I would highly recommend this book as a quick measurement reference for all those interpreting and performing ultrasound scans.

Carol A. Mittelstaedt, MD
Professor of Radiology
Department of Radiology
University of North Carolina
School of Medicine
Chapel Hill, North Carolina
USA

PREFACE

Anatomical measurements are made frequently during the course of an ultrasound examination. Measurements enable us to distinguish normal from abnormal. Many measurements are common knowledge for experienced sonographers; others are encountered less frequently, necessitating referral to textbooks. Standard ultrasound textbooks comprehensively cover the 'normal' measurements; but this information is likely to be buried in the text. Other books deal with all radiological measurement, including ultrasound, but locating the relevant information quickly may be cumbersome.

We recognized the need for a succinct, easy-to-use pocket text of ultrasound measurement when we witnessed residents, sonographers and experienced practitioners reaching for a textbook to look up a measurement. We have attempted to construct a 'pocket' textbook with easy-to-read text and good quality images to allow anyone practising ultrasound to make an accurate measurement of a normal structure. Of course many of these measurements will be frequently used in practice, while others will not. We have included the most commonly used measurements covering abdominal, pelvic, obstetric & gynaecological, pediatric, vascular, small parts and transplant imaging. This is not meant to cover all measurements used in ultrasound, but should include all those likely to be in everyday use by general sonographers or radiologists. Those requiring more specialized measurements will need to refer to the appropriate textbooks. We have not included a section on echocardiography, as this is often a specialized practice in the remit of the cardiologist.

We hope that this text will be of some use to radiology residents, sonographers in training and to the more experienced practitioner requiring a quick 'update' on a less practised measurement.

Paul S. Sidhu and Wui K. Chong

ACKNOWLEDGEMENTS

As with any book, a large number of people make contributions, which are often unacknowledged in the final manuscript. Without their contributions success would not be guaranteed.

We wish to thank Mrs. Philippa Warren for her help with typing the manuscript and offering advice as to the general layout. Special thanks to Pat Farrant for reviewing the manuscript and pointing out areas where improvements could be made.

On any book on normal measurements, a whole host of volunteers are required in order to obtain images of normal anatomy. To this effect we wish to thank Joanne Poole DCR(R), Derek Svasti-Salee MD, Ian Stanton MD, Jason Wilkins MD, Sue Rowe MD, Ashley Shaw MD, Sue Rzepka RDMS and Sergio Khomyak RDMS. In addition, thanks go to Vicky Soh's then unnamed and unborn child!

Finally (PS), thanks must go to my wife, Monica and children, Gianluca and Francesca for their remarkable tolerance.

1

ABDOMEN (LIVER, GALLBLADDER AND SPLEEN)

Keshthra Satchithananda,
Zelena A. Aziz,
Maria E.K. Sellars and
Paul S. Sidhu

Liver (adult)	2
Liver (pediatric)	4
Gallbladder (adult)	6
Gallbladder (pediatric)	8
Gallbladder (neonatal)	10
Gallbladder wall	12
Common bile duct (adult)	14
Common bile duct (pediatric)	18
Hepatic duct (adult)	20
Spleen (adult and pediatric)	22
Diaphragmatic motion	26

Liver (adult)

PREPARATION
None.

POSITION
Supine, right anterior oblique to demonstrate the porta hepatis.

PROBE
2.0–4.0 MHz curvilinear transducer.

METHOD
Longitudinal views are taken in the midclavicular and midline positions, and measurements obtained. Anteroposterior diameters are also measured at the midpoint of the longitudinal diameters. All measurements are taken on deep inspiration.

APPEARANCE
Uniform pattern of medium strength echoes.

MEASUREMENTS

Diameter	Mean ± SD (cm)
Midclavicular longitudinal	10.5 ± 1.5
Midclavicular anteroposterior	8.1 ± 1.9
Midline longitudinal	8.3 ± 1.7
Midline anteroposterior	5.7 ± 1.5

In the transverse plane, the normal caudate lobe should be less than 2/3 of the size of the right lobe.

FURTHER READING
Harbin WP, Robert NJ, Ferrucci JT. Diagnosis of cirrhosis based on regional changes in hepatic morphology: a radiological and pathological analysis. *Radiology* 1980;**135**:273–283.
Niederau C, Sonnenberg A, Muller JE, Erckenbrecht JF, Scholten T, Fritsch WP. Sonographic measurements of the normal liver, spleen, pancreas, and portal vein. *Radiology* 1983;**149**:537–540.

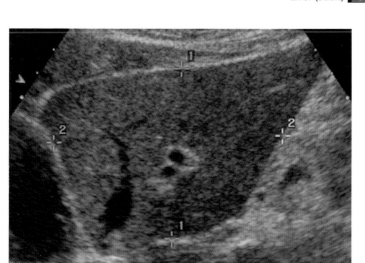

Figure 1a Longitudinal view through the left lobe of the liver obtained in the midline. Cursor 1, anteroposterior diameter; cursor 2, midline longitudinal diameter

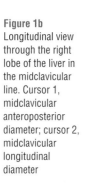

Figure 1b
Longitudinal view through the right lobe of the liver in the midclavicular line. Cursor 1, midclavicular anteroposterior diameter; cursor 2, midclavicular longitudinal diameter

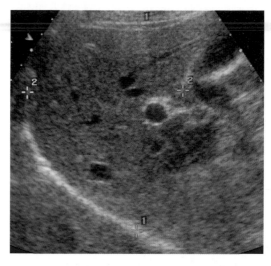

Liver (pediatric)

PREPARATION
None.

POSITION
Supine, right anterior oblique positions to demonstrate the porta hepatis.

PROBE
4.0–10.0 MHz curvilinear transducer.

METHOD
Longitudinal images of the right lobe are taken in the midclavicular or midaxillary positions. The length of the liver is measured from the uppermost portion of the dome of the diaphragm to the inferior tip.

APPEARANCE
Uniform pattern of medium strength echoes.

MEASUREMENTS

Age (months)	Length of right lobe of liver (mean ± SD, mm)
1–3	64 ± 10.4
4–6	73 ± 10.8
7–9	79 ± 8.0
12–30	85 ± 10.0
36–59	86 ± 11.8
60–83	100 ± 13.6
84–107	105 ± 10.6
108–131	105 ± 12.5
132–155	115 ± 14.0
156–179	118 ± 14.6
180–200	121 ± 11.7

FURTHER READING
Konus OL, Ozdemir A, Akkaya A, Erbas G, Celik H, Isik S. Normal liver, spleen, and kidney dimensions in neonates, infants, and children: evaluation with sonography. *American Journal of Roentgenology* 1998;**171**:1693–1698.

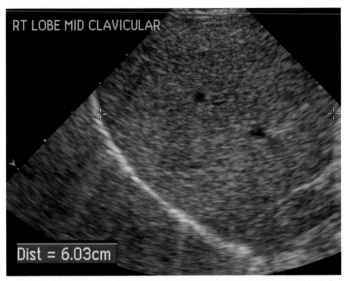

Figure 2a Longitudinal views of the right lobe in the midclavicular position with the length measured from the dome of the diaphragm to the inferior tip of the liver

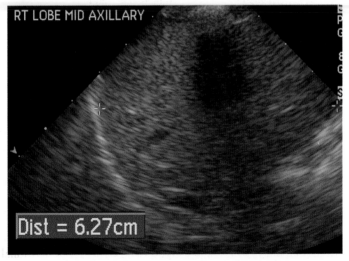

Figure 2b Longitudinal views of the right lobe in the midaxillary position with the length measured from the dome of the diaphragm to the inferior tip of the liver

Gallbladder (adult)

PREPARATION
Patient should be fasted for 6–8 hours before examination.

POSITION
The gallbladder is initially examined in the supine position. Then the patient is turned to the right anterior oblique position to ensure any small mobile stones are not missed.

PROBE
2.0–4.0 MHz curvilinear transducer.

METHOD
Longitudinal and transverse images are taken from a subcostal or an intercostal approach on deep inspiration in the supine and right anterior oblique positions.

APPEARANCE
On a longitudinal image the gallbladder appears as an echo-free pear-shaped structure. The gallbladder wall is smooth and is seen as a line of high reflectivity.

MEASUREMENTS
There is considerable variation in the size and shape of the gallbladder, but certain reference values do exist.

Length (mm)	Width (mm)
Newborn 30–32	1/3 of length
Adult 100 (range 80–120)	40–50

FURTHER READING
Carroll BA, Oppenheimer DA, Muller HH. High-frequency real-time ultrasound of the neonatal biliary system. *Radiology* 1982;**145**:437–440.

Dodds WJ, Groh WJ, Darweesh RM, Lawson TL, Kishk SM, Kern MK. Sonographic measurement of gallbladder volume. *American Journal of Roentgenology* 1985;**145**:1009–1011.

Finberg HJ, Birnholz JC. Ultrasound evaluation of the gallbladder wall. *Radiology* 1979;**133**:693–698.

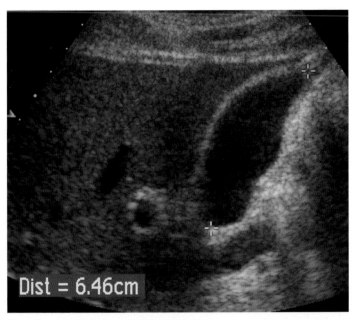

Figure 3a   Longitudinal aspect of the gallbladder

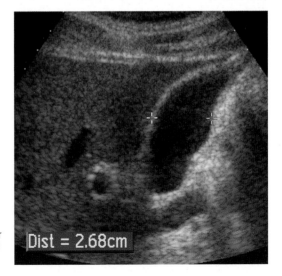

Figure 3b
Transverse diameter
at the mid aspect of
the gallbladder

Gallbladder (pediatric)

PREPARATION
Younger patients should fast for 3 hours; older children should fast for 6–8 hours before examination.

POSITION
The gallbladder is initially examined in the supine position, and then the patient is turned to right anterior oblique position.

PROBE
4.0–6.0 MHz curvilinear transducer.

METHOD
Longitudinal and transverse images are obtained from a subcostal or intercostal approach in the supine and right anterior oblique positions.

APPEARANCE
On a longitudinal image the gallbladder appears as an echo-free pear-shaped structure.

MEASUREMENTS

Age (years)	Length, mean and range (mm)	Width, mean and range (mm)
2–5	42 (29–52)	17 (14–23)
6–8	56 (44–74)	18 (10–24)
9–11	55 (34–65)	19 (12–32)
12–16	61 (38–80)	20 (13–28)

FURTHER READING
McGahan JP, Phillips HE, Cox KL. Sonography of the normal pediatric gallbladder and biliary tract. *Radiology* 1982;**144**:873–875.

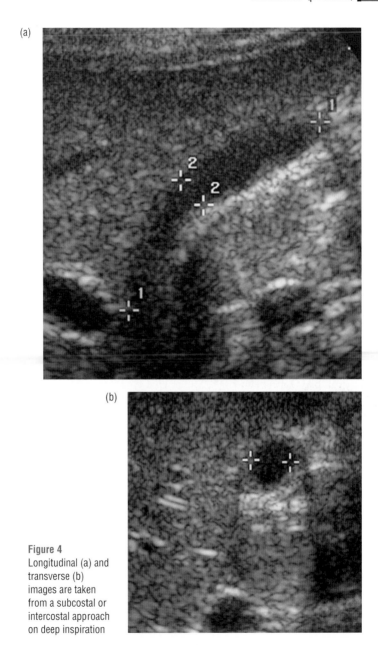

(a)

(b)

Figure 4
Longitudinal (a) and transverse (b) images are taken from a subcostal or intercostal approach on deep inspiration

Gallbladder (neonatal)

PREPARATION
Patient should not be fasted before examination.

POSITION
The gallbladder is initially examined in the supine position. Then the patient is turned to right anterior oblique position.

PROBE
8.0–13.0 MHz curvilinear transducer.

METHOD
Longitudinal and transverse images are obtained from a subcostal or intercostal approach in the supine and right anterior oblique positions.

APPEARANCE
On a longitudinal image the gallbladder appears as an echo-free pear shaped structure. The gallbladder wall is smooth and is seen as a line of high reflectivity.

MEASUREMENTS
Length 30–32 mm; width 1/3 of length.

FURTHER READING
Carroll BA, Oppenheimer DA, Muller HH. High-frequency real-time ultrasound of the neonatal biliary system. *Radiology* 1982;**145**:437–440.

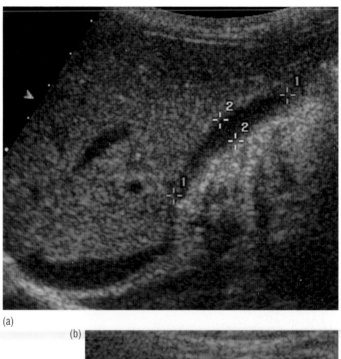

(a)

(b)

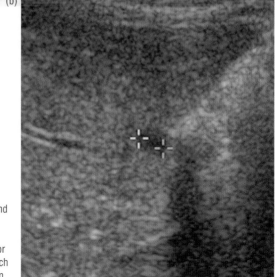

Figure 5
Longitudinal (a) and
transverse (b)
images are taken
from a subcostal or
intercostal approach
on deep inspiration

Gallbladder wall

PREPARATION
Patient should be fasted for 6–8 hours before examination.

POSITION
Supine or left lateral decubitus positions. Imaging is performed in either the longitudinal or transverse plane.

PROBE
2.0–4.0 MHz curvilinear transducer.

METHOD
Longitudinal and transverse images are taken from a subcostal or an intercostal approach on deep inspiration in the supine and left lateral decubitus positions.

APPEARANCE
On a longitudinal image the gallbladder appears as an echo-free pear-shaped structure. The gallbladder wall is smooth and is seen as a line of high reflectivity.

MEASUREMENTS
Measurement of the gallbladder wall is made along the axis of the ultrasound beam using the portion of the gallbladder contiguous with the liver and including all identifiable layers. Average wall thickness is 2–3 mm. Wall thickness greater than 3.5 mm is highly suggestive of disease. A wall thickness of 3 mm or less does not rule out cholecystitis.

FURTHER READING
Engel JM, Deitch EA, Sikkema W. Gallbladder wall thickness: sonographic accuracy and relation to disease. *American Journal of Roentgenology* 1980;**134**:907–909.

Finberg HJ, Birnholz JC. Ultrasound evaluation of the gallbladder wall. *Radiology* 1979;**13**:693–698.

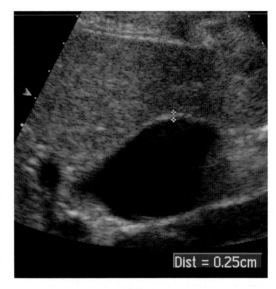

Dist = 0.25cm

Figure 6 The thickness of the gallbladder wall is measured along the long axis of the ultrasound beam in an area where the gallbladder is contiguous with the liver

Common bile duct (adult)

PREPARATION
Patient should be fasted for 6–8 hours before examination.

POSITION
Initially supine, then turn to the right anterior oblique or lateral decubitis positions to demonstrate the common duct.

PROBE
2.0–4.0 MHz curvilinear transducer.

METHOD
Patient is imaged from a subcostal position, in the longitudinal plane or from an intercostal position. The common duct is measured at a point that passes anterior to the right portal vein, often with the hepatic artery seen in cross-section between the duct and the vein. The measurement is taken from the inner wall to the inner wall and should be perpendicular to the course of the duct.

APPEARANCE
The extrahepatic bile duct may be divided into three segments: the hilar segment in front of the main portal vein, the suprapancreatic and the intrapancreatic segment which is ventral to the inferior vena cava and passes through the pancreatic head. The maximal anteroposterior diameter of the extrahepatic bile duct is measured.

MEASUREMENTS
Average measurement for a normal adult is 4 mm, though up to 6 mm is accepted as normal. The mean common duct diameter following cholecystectomy is 7.7 ± 2.1 mm. After cholecystectomy 8–10 mm can be normal. There is an age-dependent change in the diameter of the common duct and it can be up to 10 mm in the very elderly.

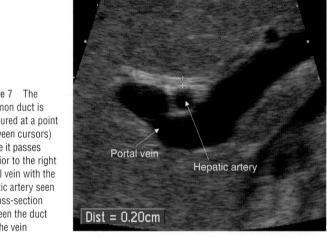

Figure 7 The common duct is measured at a point (between cursors) where it passes anterior to the right portal vein with the hepatic artery seen in cross-section between the duct and the vein

Location	Anteroposterior diameter (mean $\pm$ SD, mm)
Proximal	2.9 $\pm$ 1.1
Middle	3.5 $\pm$ 1.2
Distal	3.5 $\pm$ 1.2

Reproduced with permission from Horrow MM, Horrow JC, Niakosari A, Kirby CL, Rosenberg HK. Is age associated with size of adult extrahepatic bile duct: sonographic study. *Radiology* 2001;**221**:411–414.

Age (years)	Common bile duct size[1] (mean $\pm$ SD, mm)	
	Male	**Female**
<21	3.3 $\pm$ 1.1	3.3 $\pm$ 1.1
21–30	4.7 $\pm$ 1.3	4.7 $\pm$ 1.2
31–40	5.0 $\pm$ 1.5	4.6 $\pm$ 1.4
41–50	5.4 $\pm$ 1.4	5.3 $\pm$ 1.2
51–60	6.2 $\pm$ 1.9	5.3 $\pm$ 1.8
>60	6.1 $\pm$ 2.0	6.8 $\pm$ 1.7

The extrahepatic duct may be measured at three locations: in the porta hepatis (proximal), in the most distal aspect of the head of the pancreas (distal) and midway between these measurements.[2]

REFERENCES

1. Horrow MM, Horrow JC, Niakosari A, Kirby CL, Rosenberg HK. Is age associated with size of adult extrahepatic bile duct: sonographic study. *Radiology* 2001;**221**:411–414.
2. Wu CC, Ho YH, Chen CY. Effect of age on common bile duct diameter: a real-time ultrasonographic study. *Journal of Clinical Ultrasound* 1984;**12**:473–478.

FURTHER READING

Feng B, Song Q. Does the common bile duct dilate after cholecystectomy? *American Journal of Roentgenology* 1995;**165**:859–861.

Hunt DR, Scott AJ. Changes in bile duct diameter after cholecystectomy: A 5-year prospective study. *Gastroenterology* 1989;**97**:1485–1488.

Parulekar SG. Ultrasound evaluation of common bile duct size. *Radiology* 1979;**133**:703–707.

Common bile duct (pediatric)

PREPARATION
None.

POSITION
Initially supine, then turn to the right anterior oblique position to demonstrate the common duct.

PROBE
4.0–6.0 MHz curvilinear transducer.

METHOD
Patient is imaged from a subcostal position in the longitudinal plane or from an intercostal position. The common bile duct may be identified by means of the anatomic course within the gastroduodenal ligament, coursing distally to the head of the pancreas and absence of flow with Doppler interrogation. The internal diameter of the extrahepatic duct is measured from inner wall to inner wall.

APPEARANCE
With high resolution imaging normal intrahepatic ducts can be visualized as tubular structures with thin high-reflective walls. The term 'common duct' is used, since it is not possible on ultrasound to demonstrate the entrance of the cystic duct, and thus differentiate the common hepatic duct from the common bile duct.

MEASUREMENTS
The common duct of neonates and children younger than 1 year should be 1.6 mm or less in diameter from inner wall to inner wall. The size increases slowly with age. The common duct during childhood and early adolescence should not measure more than 2.5–3.0 mm in diameter. It is a distensible structure that demonstrates small but statistically significant changes in size during daily fluctuations in the bile flow.

FURTHER READING
Hernanz-Schulman M, Ambrosino MM, Freeman PC, Quinn CB.
    Common bile duct in children. Sonographic dimensions.
    Radiology 1995;**195**:193–195.

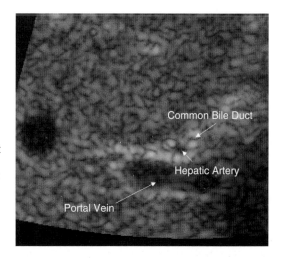

Figure 8 The common duct is measured at a point where it passes anterior to the right portal vein with the hepatic artery seen in cross-section between the duct and the vein

Hepatic duct (adult)

PREPARATION
Patient should be fasted for 6–8 hours before examination.

POSITION
Initially supine, then turn to the right anterior oblique position to demonstrate the common duct.

PROBE
2.0–4.0 MHz curvilinear transducer.

METHOD
Patient is imaged from a subcostal plane, in the longitudinal direction or from an intercostal plane.

APPEARANCE
With high resolution imaging normal intrahepatic ducts can be visualized as tubular structures with thin high-reflective walls.

MEASUREMENTS
Normal hepatic duct is measured at 3 mm internal diameter (normal hepatic ducts are under half the size of the corresponding portal vein and have a straight course).

FURTHER READING
Dewbury KC. Visualisation of normal biliary ducts with ultrasound. *British Journal of Radiology* 1980;**53**:774–780.

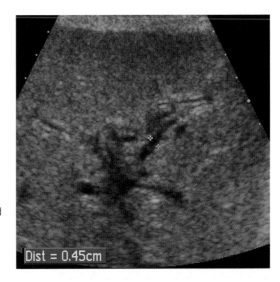

Figure 9 A dilated peripheral hepatic duct (between cursors) in the left lobe of the liver

Dist = 0.45cm

Spleen (adult and pediatric)

PREPARATION
None.

POSITION
Left upper abdomen in the midaxillary line, then turn patient to left anterior oblique position as necessary to view the spleen.

PROBE
2.0–5.0 MHz curvilinear transducer.

METHOD
Splenic length measured during quiet breathing, obtained from a coronal plane that includes the hilum. The greatest longitudinal distance between the splenic dome and the tip (splenic length) is measured. Transverse, longitudinal and diagonal diameters are measured from the image showing maximum cross-sectional area in a coronal plane.

APPEARANCE
Spleen should show a uniform homogeneous echo pattern. It is slightly less reflective than the liver.

MEASUREMENTS
Length: A measurement of length and diameter can be made in the oblique plane at the 10th and 11th intercostal space, through the splenic hilum (length ≤12 cm, diameter ≤7 cm). Spleen size correlates with height rather than age.

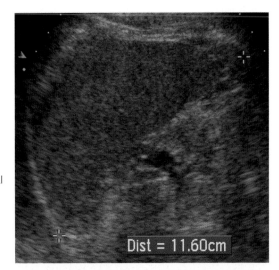

Figure 10a The greatest longitudinal distance between the splenic dome and the tip is measured as the splenic length (between cursors)

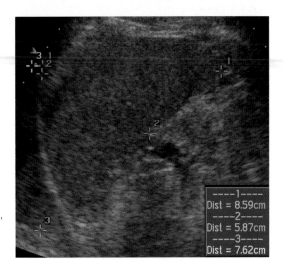

Figure 10b Three measurements are obtained (cursors 1, 2 and 3) in order to calculate splenic area

Age	Splenic length in children (cm) (North American population)[1]	
(months)	Median (10th–90th centile)	Suggested upper limit
0–3	4.5 (3.3–5.8)	6.0
3–6	5.3 (4.9–6.4)	6.5
6–12	6.2 (5.2–6.8)	7.0
(years)		
1–2	6.9 (5.4–7.5)	8.0
2–4	7.4 (6.4–8.6)	9.0
4–6	7.8 (6.9–8.8)	9.5
6–8	8.2 (7.0–9.6)	10.0
8–10	9.2 (7.9–10.5)	11.0
10–12	9.9 (8.6–10.9)	11.5
12–15	10.1 (8.7–11.4)	12.0
15–20 (male)	10.0 (9.0–11.7)	13.0
15–20 (female)	11.2 (10.1–12.6)	12.0

Age	Normal splenic lengths (Chinese population)[2]	
(years)	(mean ± SD, cm) Male	Female
0–4	5.94 ± 1.18	5.77 ± 1.21
5–9	7.81 ± 1.28	7.48 ± 1.21
10–14	9.10 ± 1.41	8.76 ± 1.10
15–19	10.04 ± 1.29	8.61 ± 1.03
20–29	9.57 ± 1.0	9.08 ± 1.26
30–39	9.52 ± 1.29	8.88 ± 1.28
40–49	9.38 ± 1.48	8.92 ± 1.54
50–59	8.83 ± 1.33	8.25 ± 1.39
60–69	8.99 ± 1.61	8.66 ± 1.50
70–79	8.60 ± 1.62	8.25 ± 1.54
80–89	7.90 ± 1.85	7.59 ± 1.53

Area: View the spleen in the longitudinal axis, in deep inspiration. The interface between lung and spleen serves as the transverse diameter and the longitudinal diameter is measured from here to the splenic tip. The diagonal diameter is measured from this lateral spleen–lung interface to the medial spleen margin. The cross-sectional area is calculated:[3]

diagonal/$\sqrt{}$ (transverse^2 + longitudinal^2)/2

Normal	Diameter (mean $\pm$ SD, cm)
Transverse diameter	5.5 ± 1.4
Longitudinal diameter	5.8 ± 1.8
Diagonal diameter	3.7 ± 1.0

REFERENCES
1. Rosenberg HK, Markowitz RI, Kolberg H, Park C, Hubbard A, Bell RD. Normal splenic size in infants and children: sonographic measurements. *American Journal of Roentgenology* 1991;**157**:119–121.
2. Loftus WK, Metreweli C. Normal splenic size in a Chinese population. *Journal of Ultrasound in Medicine* 1997;**16**:345–347.
3. Niederau C, Sonnenberg A, Muller JE, Erckenbrecht JF, Scholten T, Fritsch WP. Sonographic measurements of the normal liver, spleen, pancreas, and portal vein. *Radiology* 1983;**149**:537–540.

Diaphragmatic motion

PREPARATION
None.

POSITION
Supine.

PROBE
3.5–5.0 MHz curvilinear transducer.

METHOD
Performed from a subcostal position, in a longitudinal plane. A cursor is placed at the position of the dome of either the left or right hemi-diaphragm at end tidal volume, and then marked at full inspiration. If forced expiration is used, the dome of the diaphragm may not be visible.

APPEARANCE
The thin high-reflective diaphragmatic curve is readily identified.

MEASUREMENTS
The estimated diaphragmatic movements for adults are:
- deep inspiration   5.4 cm (male), 4.0 cm (female)
- quiet inspiration   2.2 cm

FURTHER READING
Harris RS, Giovannetti M, Kim BK. Normal ventilatory movement of the right hemidiaphragm studied by ultrasonography and pneumotachoraphy. *Radiology* 1983;**146**:141–144.

Houston JG, Morris AD, Howie CA, Reid JL, McMillan N. Technical report: quantitative assessment of diaphragmatic movement – a reproducible method using ultrasound. *Clinical Radiology* 1992;**46**:40–407.

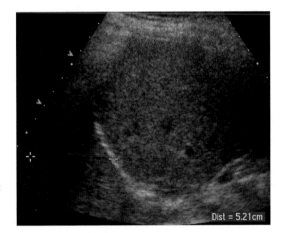

Figure 11 A cursor is placed at the position of the dome of the right hemidiaphragm at end tidal volume, and then marked at full inspiration with a further cursor

Dist = 5.21 cm

2 ABDOMEN (VASCULAR)

Zelena A. Aziz,
Keshthra Satchithananda and
Paul S. Sidhu

Renal artery	30
Evaluation of acute renal obstruction with intrarenal Doppler	34
Portal vein	36
Hepatic veins	38
Hepatic artery	40
Celiac and superior mesenteric arteries	42
Doppler ultrasound measurement of postprandial intestinal blood flow	46
Inferior mesenteric artery	48

Renal artery

PREPARATION
None.

POSITION
Supine, lateral decubitus and if necessary prone positions.

PROBE
2.0–5.0 MHz curvilinear transducer.

METHOD
The origin of the renal arteries may be visualized using the liver/spleen as an acoustic window in the oblique positions. Spectral Doppler waveforms are obtained from proximal, mid and distal sites within the main renal artery and from interlobar or segmental vessels in the upper, mid and lower poles. The Doppler angle should be kept as close to 60° as possible.

MEASUREMENTS
Renal–aortic ratio (RAR): Determined using the highest peak systolic velocity from the renal artery divided by the peak systolic velocity in the aorta. RAR of >3.0 is a reliable predictor of renal artery stenosis of ≥60%, and >3.5 indicates 60–99% stenosis.

Peak systolic velocity (PSV): PSV of >180 cm/s is a predictor of renal artery stenosis ≥60%.

Resistance index (RI):

   RI = (peak systolic velocity – end systolic velocity)/peak systolic velocity

The RI value of the normal right and left kidney is 0.60 and 0.59 respectively. There is variability of measurements within a kidney, and a number of RI values should be averaged before a single representative value is reported. In renal artery stenosis (RAS), the RI is measured in the interlobar arteries.

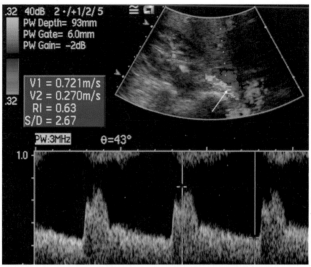

Figure 12a An oblique view through the right kidney demonstrates the renal artery arising from the aorta (arrow). A peak systolic velocity of 0.72 m/s is obtained from the proximal aspect of the renal artery

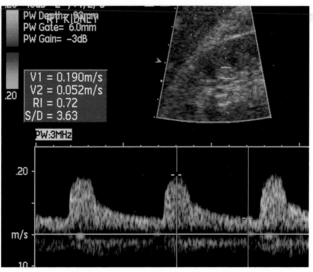

Figure 12b The resistance index is measured as 0.72 in an interlobar segmental vessel in the right kidney

Mean RI for control group and in RAS[1]

	Controls	**RAS >70%**
Mean ± SD	0.64 ± 0.07	0.49 ± 0.14
Range	0.47–0.80	0.32–0.71

A RI >0.70 in the native kidney is indicative of abnormal renovascular resistance.

REFERENCE
1. Schwerk WB, Restrepo IK, Klose KJ, Schade-Brittinger C. Renal artery stenosis: grading with image-directed Doppler US evaluation of renal resistive index. *Radiology* 1994;**190**:785–790.

FURTHER READING
House MK, Dowling RJ, King P, Gibson RN. Using Doppler sonography to reveal renal artery stenosis: An evaluation of optimal imaging parameters. *American Journal of Roentgenology* 1999;**173**:761–765.

Keogan MT, Kliewer MA, Hertzberg BS, DeLong DM, Tupler RH, Carroll BA. Renal resistive indexes: variability in Doppler US measurement in a healthy population. *Radiology* 1996;**199**:165–169.

Olin JW, Piedmonte MR, Young JR, DeAnna S, Grubb M, Childs MB. The utility of duplex ultrasound scanning of the renal arteries for diagnosing significant renal artery stenosis. *Annals of Internal Medicine* 1995;**122**:833–838.

Evaluation of acute renal obstruction with intrarenal Doppler

PREPARATION
None.

POSITION
Supine.

PROBE
3.5–5.0 MHz curvilinear transducer.

METHOD
Doppler signals are obtained from arcuate arteries at the corticomedullary junction or interlobar arteries along the border of medullary pyramids. The Doppler waveforms should be made on the lowest pulse repetition frequency without aliasing to maximize the size of the Doppler spectrum. The resistance index (RI) is calculated from the formula:

RI = (peak systolic velocity – end diastolic velocity)/peak systolic velocity

APPEARANCE
The normal spectral Doppler waveforms in the renal arcuate arteries are those of a low-resistance end-organ, with a broad systolic peak and an elevated end-diastolic velocity.

MEASUREMENTS
Mean RI in normal kidneys is 0.60 ± 0.04.
Mean RI of obstructed kidneys is 0.77 ± 0.07.
Elevation of the RI occurs after just 6 hours of clinical obstruction. If there is pyelosinus extravasation on the intravenous urogram (IVU) or the duration of obstruction is less than 6 hours, the RI may not be elevated.

FURTHER READING
Platt JF, Rubin JM, Ellis JH. Acute renal obstruction: evaluation with intrarenal duplex Doppler and conventional US. *Radiology* 1993;**186**:685–688.
Rodgers PM, Bates JA, Irving HC. Intrarenal Doppler studies in normal and acutely obstructed kidneys. *British Journal of Radiology* 1992;**65**:207–212.

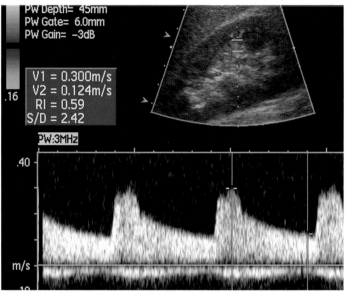

Figure 13 Doppler signals are obtained from arcuate arteries at the corticomedullary junction or interlobar arteries along the border of medullary pyramids. The resistance index is calculated from the spectral Doppler waveform obtained

Portal vein

PREPARATION
Fasting for 4–6 hours.

POSITION
Supine and right anterior oblique.

PROBE
2.0–5.0 MHz curvilinear transducer.

METHOD
Right longitudinal intercostal approach.

MEASUREMENTS
Normal portal venous velocity varies in the same individual, increasing after a meal and decreasing after exercise. The diameter is measured at the broadest point just distal to union of splenic and superior mesenteric vein, normally measuring 11 ± 2 mm. Color and spectral Doppler imaging demonstrates the portal venous system to be an isolated vascular unit with a relatively monophasic flow pattern with fluctuations with cardiac or respiratory movements. The Valsalva maneuver results in portal vein dilatation. The normal portal vein velocity is 14–18 cm/s (angle of insonation $\leq 60°$).

Congestion index (CI) of the portal vein:

portal vein area = diameter A × diameter B × $\pi/4$
flow velocity = $0.57 \times$ maximum portal vein velocity (angle $\leq 60°$)
CI = portal vein area/flow velocity

The normal value for the CI is 0.070 ± 0.029 cm/s and increases to 0.171 ± 0.075 cm/s in patients with cirrhosis.

FURTHER READING
Moriyasu F, Nishida O, Ban N, Nakamura T, Sakai M, Miyake T, Uchino H. 'Congestion Index' of the portal vein. *American Journal of Roentgenology* 1986;**146**:735–739.

Weinreb J, Kumari S, Phillips G; Pochaczevsky R. Portal vein measurements by real time sonography. *American Journal of Roentgenology* 1982;**139**:497–499.

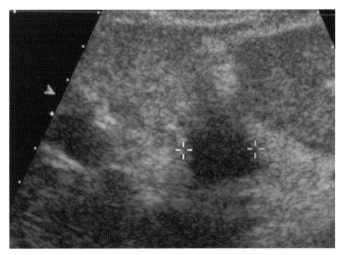

Figure 14a   The diameter of the portal vein is measured at the broadest point just distal to the union of the splenic and superior mesenteric vein

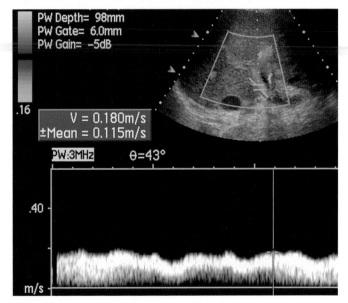

Figure 14b   A spectral Doppler waveform obtained from the portal vein demonstrates a relatively monophasic flow pattern

Hepatic veins

PREPARATION
None.

POSITION
Supine and right anterior oblique.

PROBE
2.0–5.0 MHz curvilinear transducer.

METHOD
Right lateral intercostal approach during quiet respiration. Place spectral Doppler gate halfway along length of the hepatic vein.

APPEARANCES
There are usually three main hepatic veins (left, middle and right) but many patients have an accessory or inferior right hepatic vein. These join centrally into the IVC immediately inferior to the diaphragm. Pulsatility within left hepatic vein is greater than the middle vein, which is greater than the right vein, due to transmitted pulsations from heart. To minimize this effect, the right hepatic vein is normally used for Doppler studies.

MEASUREMENTS
Doppler spectral flow shows a triphasic waveform with two periods of forward flow within each cardiac cycle (corresponding to the two phases of right atrial filling) and the one period of normal, transient reversed flow due to contraction of the right side of the heart. This triphasic pattern alters in cirrhosis, becoming biphasic and eventually monophasic in advanced disease. Pattern alterations are also observed in heart failure and tricuspid regurgitation.

FURTHER READING
Abu-Yousef MM. Duplex Doppler sonography of the hepatic vein in tricuspid regurgitation. *American Journal of Roentgenology* 1991;**156**:79–83.

Bolondi L, Li Bassi S, Gaiani S, Zironi G, Benzi G, Santi V, Barbara L. Liver cirrhosis: changes of Doppler waveform of hepatic veins. *Radiology* 1991;**178**:513–516.

Farrant P, Meire HB. Hepatic vein pulsatility assessment on spectral Doppler ultrasound (short communication). *British Journal of Radiology* 1997;**70**:829–832.

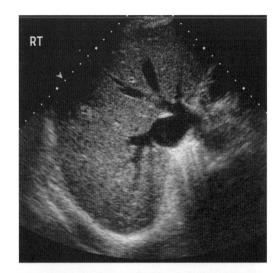

Figure 15a
Transverse
subcostal view
demonstrates the
hepatic veins
draining into the
inferior vena cava

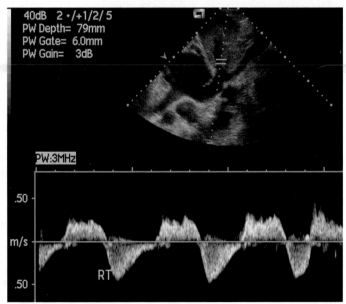

Figure 15b   A spectral Doppler gate placed over a hepatic vein demonstrates the
normal triphasic waveform with two periods of forward flow and one period of
transient reversed flow, within each cardiac cycle

Hepatic artery

PREPARATION
None.

POSITION
Supine and right anterior oblique.

PROBE
2.0–5.0 MHz curvilinear transducer.

METHOD
Right oblique intercostal approach. Locate the celiac axis anterior to aorta and then follow arterial branch that runs to the right.

APPEARANCES
The hepatic artery originates as one of the three major branches of the celiac axis, lying anteromedial to the portal vein at the porta hepatis. In 50% there is some anatomic variation or aberrant origin of the artery, either an accessory or more commonly a replaced artery. On the right, the superior mesenteric artery most commonly gives rise to the aberrant artery, often dorsal to the portal vein.

MEASUREMENTS
Resistance index (RI): Measured as proper hepatic artery crosses portal vein.

RI = (peak systolic velocity – end diastolic velocity)/peak systolic velocity

The RI of the normal hepatic artery is 0.62 ± 0.04 and can alter significantly after a 'standard' meal, increasing to 0.66–0.78.

Doppler perfusion index (DPI): DPI of the hepatic artery, which is elevated in the presence of colorectal hepatic metastases, may be calculated as follows:

DPI = hepatic arterial flow/total liver blood flow
where total liver blood flow = hepatic arterial blood flow + portal venous blood flow; blood flow = time-average velocity of blood vessel × time-average cross sectional area of lumen of vessel.

The upper limit of normal range of DPI is 0.25.

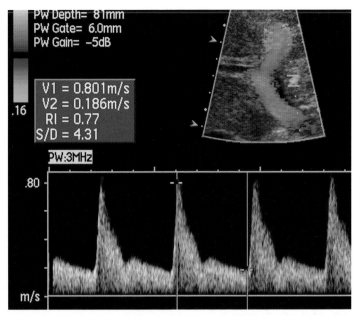

Figure 16 The hepatic artery is located adjacent to the portal vein and a spectral Doppler gate identifies the low-resistance waveform pattern

FURTHER READING

Grant EG, Schiller VL, Millener P, Tessler FN, Perrella RR, Ragavendra N, Busuttil R. Color Doppler imaging of the hepatic vasculature. *American Journal of Roentgenology* 1992;**159**:943–950.

Joynt LK, Platt JF, Rubin JM, Ellis JH, Bude RO. Hepatic artery resistance before and after standard meal. Subjects with diseased and healthy livers. *Radiology* 1995;**196**:489–492.

Leen E, Goldberg JA, Robertson J, Angerson WJ, Sutherland GR, Cooke TG, McArdle CS. Early detection of occult colorectal metastases using duplex colour Doppler sonography. *British Journal of Surgery* 1993;**80**:1249–1251.

Celiac and superior mesenteric arteries

PREPARATION
Ultrasound performed after an 8–12 hour fast.

POSITION
Patient supine with head of bed elevated 30°.

PROBE
2.0–4.0 MHz curvilinear transducer.

METHOD
Ensure Doppler angle of ≤60°. Locate the level of the suprarenal aorta in the transverse plane, identifying the celiac artery (CA) and the superior mesenteric artery (SMA), and then examine in the longitudinal direction. Measure the peak systolic velocity (PSV) a few centimeters from the origins.

APPEARANCE
Best seen in the longitudinal view, where the celiac axis and superior mesenteric arteries arise from the anterior aspect of the aorta, in close proximity to each other. Only high-grade mesenteric artery lesions are likely to be symptomatic; **therefore it is only important to detect stenosis of >70%.**

MEASUREMENTS

	Velocity (mean ± SD, cm/s)	
	SMA	**Celiac axis**
Normal	125 ± 25	123 ± 27
Atherosclerotic (normal on arteriography)	163 ± 59	138 ± 38
Stenosis (70–99%)	PSV ≥275	PSV ≥200

Unlike in renal artery stenosis, the velocity ratios of SMA and CA PSV to aortic PSV does not offer any advantage in the detection of 70–99% stenotic lesions. A PSV of ≥275 cm/s in the SMA or ≥200 cm/s in the CA, or no flow within a well-visualized segment of splachnic artery, accurately predicts 70–99% mesenteric stenosis or occlusion respectively.

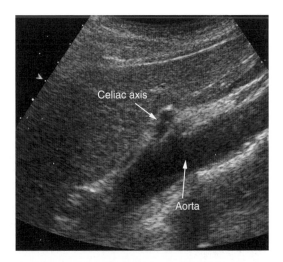

Figure 17a The celiac axis (arrow) is identified in the longitudinal section through the plane of the aorta (arrow)

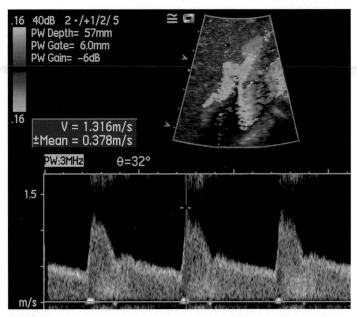

Figure 17b The peak systolic velocity is measured at 1.32 m/s in this example

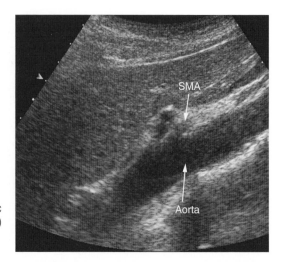

Figure 18a
Longitudinal view through the superior mesenteric artery (SMA, arrow) in the plane of the aorta (arrow)

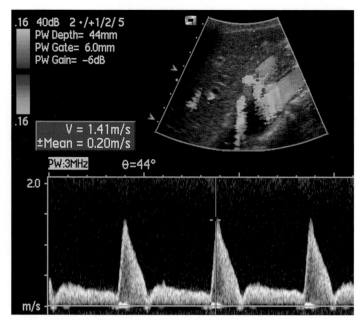

Figure 18b A spectral Doppler gate placed over the artery to record a peak systolic velocity of 1.41 m/s

FURTHER READING

Moneta GL, Yeager RA, Dalman R, Antonovic R, Hall LD, Porter
JM. Duplex ultrasound criteria for diagnosis of splanchic artery
stenosis or occlusion. *Journal of Vascular Surgery*
1991;**14**:511–520.

Doppler ultrasound measurement of postprandial intestinal blood flow

PREPARATION
Patients fast overnight and the examination is performed after 30 minutes of supine rest.

POSITION
Patient supine with head of bed elevated 30°.

PROBE
2.0–5.0 MHz curvilinear transducer.

METHOD
Superior mesenteric and celiac arteries can be identified either longitudinally or transversely. Angle of insonation kept at ≤60°, and the vessels examined along their visible length. The following parameters are measured: peak systolic velocity (PSV), end diastolic velocity (EDV) and pulsatility index (PI). A 'standard' 800 kcal (3.35 MJ) meal is consumed and serial Doppler measurements are made over the following hour.

PI = (peak systolic velocity − end diastolic velocity)/mean velocity

APPEARANCE
Best seen in the longitudinal view, where the celiac axis and superior mesenteric arteries arise from the anterior aspect of the aorta, in close proximity to each other.

MEASUREMENTS

Normal values	Before meal			After meal		
	PSV	EDV	PI	PSV	EDV	PI
	(cm/s)	(cm/s)		(cm/s)	(cm/s)	
Superior mesenteric artery	100	16	3.6	154	46	1.8
Celiac axis	120	30	1.5	130	40	1.5

A meal should cause an increase in both systolic and diastolic velocities and a reduction in the PI, indicative of a fall in distal mesenteric vascular impedance. The increase in superior mesenteric artery EDV can be

150–300%. Changes in the celiac artery are less noticeable as the bulk of celiac blood flow is not to the gut.

FURTHER READING

Muller AF. Role of duplex Doppler ultrasound in the assessment of patients with postprandial abdominal pain. *Gut* 1992;**33**:460–465.

Figure 19a Longitudinal section through the aorta to demonstrate the superior mesenteric artery (SMA, arrow)

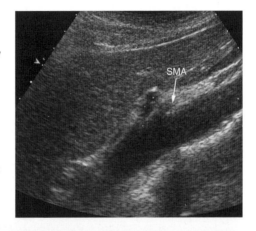

Figure 19b The spectral Doppler waveform pattern has altered following a meal, with a high forward diastolic flow (compare with image 18b, page 44)

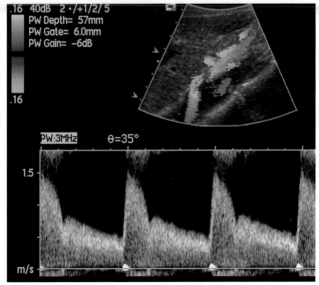

Inferior mesenteric artery

PREPARATION
Overnight fast.

POSITION
Supine.

PROBE
3.5–5.0 MHz curvilinear transducer or 7.5 MHz linear array transducer.

METHOD
The inferior mesenteric artery is identified arising from the aorta ante-riorly and to the left, spectral Doppler waveforms are obtained from the proximal 3–4 cm of the artery along its longitudinal axis (Doppler angle ≤60°). The inferior mesenteric artery is seen in 92% of subjects.

APPEARANCE
The spectral Doppler waveform often but not always demonstrates flow that tends to be triphasic with an initial high-velocity forward component during systole, followed by reversal of flow for a short duration, then low-velocity forward flow during diastole.

MEASUREMENTS

	Mean ± SD
Peak systolic velocity (PSV)	0.98 ± 0.30 m/s
End diastolic velocity (EDV)	0.11 ± 0.05 m/s
Mean velocity (V_{mean})	0.25 ± 0.08 m/s
Resistance index (RI)	0.89 ± 0.06
Pulsatility index (PI)	4.50 ± 1.53

RI = (peak systolic velocity – end diastolic velocity)/peak systolic velocity

PI = (peak systolic velocity – end diastolic velocity)/mean velocity

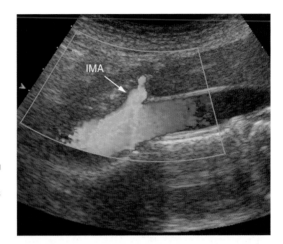

Figure 20a A longitudinal section through the lower aorta demonstrates the origin of the inferior mesenteric artery (IMA, arrow)

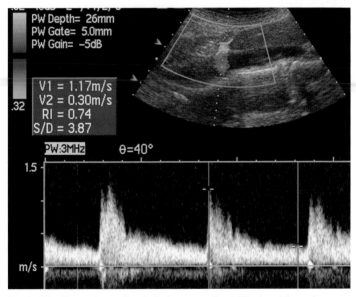

Figure 20b The peak systolic velocity is measured at 1.17 m/s and the end diastolic velocity at 0.30 m/s, giving a resistance index of 0.74

FURTHER READING

Denys AL, Lafortune M, Aubin B, Burke M, Breton G. Doppler sonography of the inferior mesenteric artery: a preliminary study. *Journal of Ultrasound in Medicine* 1995;**14**:435–439.

Erden A, Yurdakul M, Cumhur T. Doppler waveforms of the normal and collateralized inferior mesenteric artery. *American Journal of Roentgenology* 1998;**171**:619–627.

3 RETROPERITONEUM

Zelena A. Aziz,
Keshthra Satchithananda,
Maria E.K. Sellars and
Paul S. Sidhu

Kidneys (adult)	52
Kidney size (pediatric)	56
Kidney size (infant and neonatal)	60
Renal pelvic diameter (neonatal and fetal)	64
Adrenal glands (adult)	66
Adrenal glands (infant)	67
Adrenal glands (neonatal)	68
Pancreas (adult)	70
Pancreatic duct (adult)	72
Pancreas (pediatric)	74
Psoas muscle	76
Retroperitoneal lymph nodes	78

Kidneys (adult)

PREPARATION
None.

POSITION
Supine, left and right anterior oblique and if necessary, prone.

PROBE
3.5–5.0 MHz curvilinear transducer.

METHOD
Image the right kidney using the liver as an acoustic window. The left kidney is typically more difficult to visualize. The left anterior oblique 45° or right decubitus position may help, and requesting the patient to suspend respiration ensures less movement. Both kidneys should be imaged in both longitudinal and transverse planes.

APPEARANCE
The reflectivity of the renal cortex is less than the adjacent liver and spleen. The renal capsule can be identified as a thin high-reflective rim. The renal pyramids are poorly defined structures seen at the outer edge of the renal sinus. The renal sinus contains multiple structures – the pelvis, calyces, vessels and fat – and is usually of high reflectivity.

MEASUREMENTS
Three measurements are made:

Length: Obtained from the sagittal image, measuring the longest craniocaudal length.

Anteroposterior dimension: Measured from the sagittal image measured perpendicular to the long axis.

Width: Measured from a transverse image taken from the lateral margin of the kidney through the renal hilum.

Renal length decreases with age, almost entirely as a result of parenchymal reduction. Height and age but not sex are determinants of renal size. There is no difference in kidney length measurements in the supine oblique and prone positions.

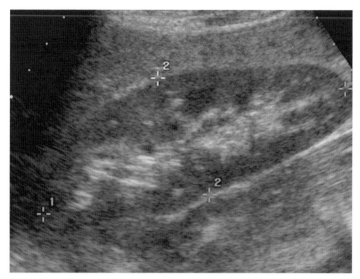

Figure 21a On the sagittal view two measurements are obtained, in the longitudinal and anteroposterior planes

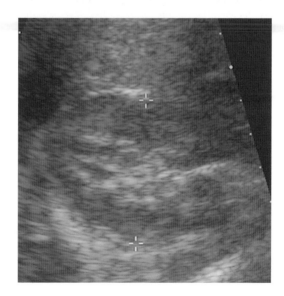

Figure 21b The width is measured from a transverse image obtained through the renal hilum

Kidney	Position	Normal values[1] (mean ± SD, cm)		
		Length	Anteroposterior	Width
Right	Oblique	10.65 ± 1.4	3.95 ± 0.8	4.92 ± 0.6
	Prone	10.74 ± 1.4	4.17 ± 0.5	5.05 ± 0.8
Left	Oblique	10.13 ± 1.2	3.58 ± 0.9	5.30 ± 0.7
	Prone	11.10 ± 1.2	4.14 ± 0.8	5.30 ± 0.8

Kidney	Size (cm) and age (decades)[2]						
	3rd	4th	5th	6th	7th	8th	9th
Right	11.3	11.2	11.2	11.0	10.7	9.9	9.6
Left	11.5	11.5	11.4	11.3	10.9	10.2	9.8

REFERENCES

1. Brandt TD, Nieman HL, Dragowski MJ, Bulawa W, Claykamp G. Ultrasound assessment of normal renal dimension. *Journal of Ultrasound in Medicine* 1982;**1**:49–52.
2. Miletic D, Fuckar Z, Sustic A, Mozetic V, Stimac D, Zauhar G. Sonographic measurement of absolute and relative renal length in adults. *Journal of Clinical Ultrasound* 1998;**26**:185–189.

FURTHER READING

Emamian SA, Nielsen MB, Pedersen JF, Ytte L. Kidney dimensions at sonography: correlation with age, sex, and habitus in 665 adult volunteers. *American Journal of Roentgenology* 1993;**160**:83–86.

Kidney size (pediatric)

PREPARATION
None.

POSITION
The prone position is useful in children.

PROBE
4.0–6.0 MHz curvilinear transducer.

METHOD
Image the right kidney using the liver as an acoustic window. The left kidney is usually more difficult to visualize. The left anterior oblique 45° or right decubitus position may help. Both kidneys must be imaged in both longitudinal and transverse planes.

APPEARANCE
The reflectivity of the renal cortex is less than the adjacent liver and spleen. The renal capsule can be identified as a thin high-reflective rim. The renal pyramids are poorly defined structures seen at the outer edge of the renal sinus. The renal sinus contains multiple structures – the pelvis, calyces, vessels and fat – and is usually of high reflectivity.

MEASUREMENTS
Measurements of kidney size are taken in the maximum longitudinal plane. In children, the length of kidneys correlates best to height,[1] although charts against age[2] and weight[1] are available. Differences between the left and right kidney are minimal.

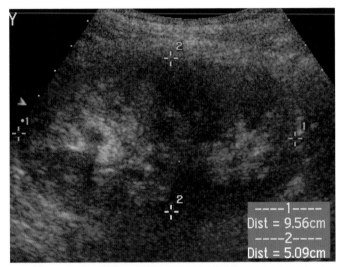

Figure 22a On the sagittal view two measurements are obtained, in the longitudinal and anteroposterior planes

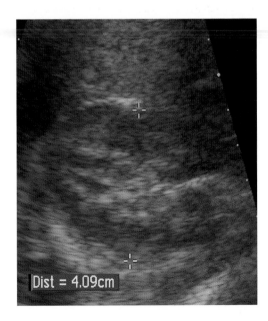

Figure 22b The width is measured from a transverse image obtained through the renal hilum

Body height (cm)	Kidney lengths[3] (mean ± SD, cm)	
	Right kidney	Left kidney
48–64	5.0 ± 0.58	5.0 ± 0.55
54–73	5.3 ± 0.53	5.6 ± 0.55
65–78	5.9 ± 0.52	6.1 ± 0.46
71–92	6.1 ± 0.34	6.6 ± 0.53
85–109	6.7 ± 0.51	7.1 ± 0.45
100–130	7.4 ± 0.55	7.9 ± 0.59
110–131	8.0 ± 0.66	8.4 ± 0.66
124–149	8.0 ± 0.70	8.4 ± 0.74
137–153	8.9 ± 0.62	9.1 ± 0.84
143–168	9.4 ± 0.59	9.6 ± 0.89
152–175	9.2 ± 0.70	9.9 ± 0.75

REFERENCES
1. Dinkel E, Erkel M, Dittrich M, Peters H, Berres M, Schulte-Wissermann H. Kidney size in childhood. Sonographical growth charts for kidney length and volume. *Pediatric Radiology* 1985;**15**:38–43.
2. Rosenbaum DM, Korngold E, Teele RL. Sonographic assessment of renal length in normal children. *American Journal of Roentgenology* 1984;**142**:467–469.
3. Konus OL, Ozdemir A, Akkaya A, Erbas G, Celik H, Isik S. Normal liver, spleen, and kidney dimensions in neonates, infants, and children: evaluation with sonography. *American Journal of Roentgenology* 1998;**171**:1693–1698.

Kidney size (infant and neonatal)

PREPARATION
None.

POSITION
Supine.

PROBE
5.0–8.0 MHz curvilinear transducer.

METHOD
Image the right kidney using the liver as an acoustic window. The left kidney is usually more difficult to visualize. The left anterior oblique 45° or right decubitus position may help. Both kidneys must be imaged in both longitudinal and transverse planes.

APPEARANCE
Accentuated corticomedullary differentiation is a normal finding in neonates and infants (age 1 day to 6 months). The medullary pyramids are seen as low-reflective triangles arranged in circular fashion around the central echogenic renal sinus; the renal cortex has higher reflectivity.

MEASUREMENTS

| | Renal lengths in term newborn infants[1] (mean ± SD, mm) | |
	Right kidney	Left kidney
Male	41.2 ± 4.4	42.7 ± 4.8
Female	41.8 ± 3.2	42.7 ± 3.7

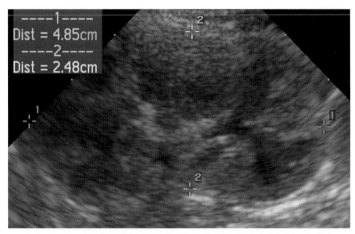

Figure 23a On the sagittal view two measurements are obtained, in the longitudinal and anteroposterior planes

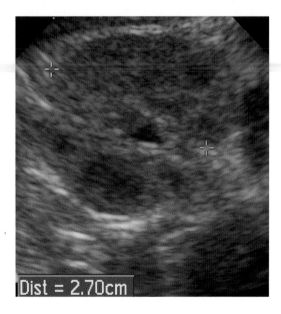

Figure 23b The width is measured from a transverse image obtained through the renal hilum

Birth weight (g)	Renal length in preterm newborn infants[2] (range, mm)
600	26.4–35.7
1000	29.4–38.7
1500	33.1–42.5
2000	36.9–46.2
2500	40.6–49.9
3000	44.3–53.7

REFERENCES

1. Holloway H, Jones TB, Robinson AE, Harpen MD, Wiseman AJ. Sonographic determination of renal volumes in normal neonates. *Pediatric Radiology* 1983;**13**:212–214.
2. Schlesinger AE, Hedlund GL, Pierson WP, Null DM. Normal standards for kidney length in premature infants: determination with US. Work in progress. *Radiology* 1987;**164**:127–129.

FURTHER READING

Haller JO, Berdon WE, Friedman AP. Increased renal cortical echogenicity: a normal finding in neonates and infants. *Radiology* 1982;**142**:173–174.

Renal pelvic diameter (neonatal and fetal)

PREPARATION
None.

POSITION
Prone.

PROBE
5.0–8.0 MHz curvilinear transducer.

METHOD
The maximum pelvic diameter is measured from transverse images.

APPEARANCE
The central reflectivity from the renal sinus fat is less prominent than in the adult and the cortex is isoreflective to the normal liver. The medullary pyramids are larger and of lower reflectivity, resulting in better corticomedullary differentiation than in the adult. Normally only a small amount of fluid is present in the renal pelvis; any dilation of the calyces is abnormal.

MEASUREMENTS
This remains a controversial area, and individual institutions will have their own protocol; the following measurements are a guide. The pelvic diameter measurements during antenatal imaging thought to represent groups at risk for significant renal abnormality are:

5 mm	at 15–20 weeks
8 mm	at 20–30 weeks
10 mm	>30 weeks

Infants with antenatal renal dilatation should have an ultrasound 1 week after birth to evaluate for severe obstruction. In infants not requiring immediate intervention or surgery for severe obstruction, repeat ultrasound and a voiding cystourethrogram is suggested at 6 weeks. If at 6 weeks the renal pelvis is less than 6 mm and there is no vesicoureteric reflux, than no further investigation is needed. If the renal pelvis is 11 mm or greater, with caliectasis, further investigation is necessary. If the renal pelvis is between 6–10 mm, then serial ultrasound examinations are suggested until the renal pelvis appears normal (<6 mm), or warrants further studies for obstruction (when >10 mm with caliectasis).

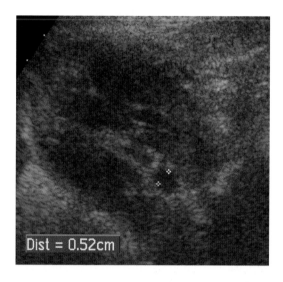

Figure 24 The maximum pelvic diameter is measured from transverse images at the point where the pelvis is at the brim of renal tissue

Dist = 0.52cm

FURTHER READING

Clautice-Engle T, Anderson NG, Allan RB, Abbott GD. Diagnosis of obstructive hydronephrosis in infants. Comparison sonograms performed 6 days and 6 weeks after birth. *American Journal of Roentgenology* 1995;**164**;963–967.

Mandell J, Blyth BR, Peters CA, Retik AB, Estroff JA, Benacerraf BR. Structural genitourinary defects detected in utero. *Radiology* 1991;**178**;193–196.

Adrenal glands (adult)

PREPARATION
None.

POSITION
Supine.

PROBE
2.0–5.0 MHz curvilinear transducer.

METHOD
Anterior transverse images in quiet respiration.

APPEARANCE
Variable appearance. An adrenal mass appears as homogeneous area with a distinct capsule. The frequencies of imaging normal adrenal glands are: 78.5% on the right and 44% on the left.

MEASUREMENTS[1]

Thickness	0.3–0.6 cm
Length	4–6 cm
Width	2–3 cm

REFERENCE
1. Yeh HC. Sonography of the adrenal glands: Normal glands and small masses. *American Journal of Roentgenology* 1980;**135**:1167–1177.

Adrenal glands (infant)

PREPARATION
None.

POSITION
Supine.

PROBE
6.0–7.5 MHz curvilinear transducer.

METHOD
Image from flanks in sagittal, coronal and transverse planes.

APPEARANCE
Thin high-reflective core representing the cortex, surrounded by a rim of low reflectivity representing the medulla. At 2 months, the cortex gets smaller and the medulla larger in proportion. At 5–6 months the whole gland is smaller, and generally of high reflectivity. At the age of 12 months, the gland is similar to the adult gland and becomes low-reflective.

MEASUREMENTS
Length is measured as maximum cephalocaudal dimension, from the apex to the base of the gland. The maximum transverse and antero-posterior diameters are measured in a transverse plane perpendicular to the length of one of the wings.

Day	Serial adrenal measurements in neonates[1] (mean $\pm$ SD, mm)		
	Transverse	Anteroposterior	Length
1	17.9 ± 2.7	9.6 ± 2.1	17.3 ± 1.8
3	14.8 ± 3.3	7.5 ± 2.2	12.8 ± 3.2
5	13.7 ± 2.1	6.9 ± 1.6	11.4 ± 2.7
11	11.8 ± 2.5	5.9 ± 1.4	8.9 ± 2.0
21	10.8 ± 1.9	5.6 ± 0.5	8.2 ± 1.2
42	9.5 ± 1.5	5.7 ± 1.0	7.7 ± 0.9

REFERENCE
1. Scott EM, Thomas A, McGarrigle HH, Lachelin GC. Serial adrenal ultrasonography in normal neonates. *Journal of Ultrasound in Medicine* 1990;9:279–283.

Adrenal glands (neonatal)

PREPARATION
None.

POSITION
Supine.

PROBE
6.0–7.5 MHz curvilinear transducer.

METHOD
Image from flanks in sagittal, coronal and transverse planes.

APPEARANCE
The adrenals have an oval shape in the transverse plane and an inverted Y-shape in the longitudinal plane. A rim of low reflectivity surrounds the thin high-reflective core. The right gland is seen in 97% and the left gland in 83%.

MEASUREMENTS
Length is measured as maximum cephalocaudal dimension. Width is maximum dimension perpendicular to the length of one of the wings.

DIMENSIONS
Length is measured as maximum cephalocaudal dimension, from the apex to the base of the gland. The maximum transverse and antero-posterior diameters are measured in a transverse plane perpendicular to the length of one of the wings. The size of the adrenal gland diminishes rapidly in the first 6 weeks of postnatal life.

Gestational age (weeks)	Mean adrenal length[1] (mm)
25–30	12
31–35	14
36–40	17

REFERENCE
1. Oppenheimer DA, Carroll BA, Yousem S. Sonography of the normal neonatal adrenal gland. *Radiology* 1983;**146**:157–160.

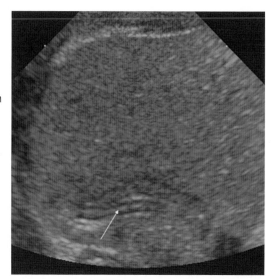

Figure 25 The adrenal gland is represented by a thin high reflective core (arrow) surrounded by a rim of low reflectivity. Length is measured as maximum cephalocaudal dimension and the width is maximum dimension perpendicular to the length of one of the wings

Pancreas (adult)

PREPARATION
None.

POSITION
Supine.

PROBE
2.0–4.0 MHz curvilinear transducer.

METHOD
If the pancreas is obscured by air, visualization may be improved by drinking 500 ml of water in the right decubitus position. The water bolus outlines the pancreatic head. Longitudinal and transverse images are obtained using the upper abdominal blood vessels as landmarks.
- The **pancreatic head** is measured above the inferior vena cava.
- The **pancreatic neck** is measured over the superior mesenteric vein.
- The **pancreatic body** is measured over the superior mesenteric artery.

APPEARANCE
The pancreas should appear homogenous with a reflectivity greater than or equal to adjacent liver. Variations in reflectivity relate to the degree of fatty infiltration. After 60 years of age, fatty accumulation in pancreatic tissues is common and reflectivity therefore increases.

MEASUREMENTS[1]

	Longitudinal (mean ± SD, cm)	Transverse (mean ± SD, cm)
Head	2.01 ± 0.39	2.08 ± 0.40
Body	1.18 ± 0.36	1.16 ± 0.29
Neck	1.00 ± 0.30	0.95 ± 0.26

Reproduced with permission from de Graaff CS, Taylor KJ, Simonds BD, Rosenfield AJ. Gray-scale echography of the pancreas. *Radiology* 1978;**129**:157–161.

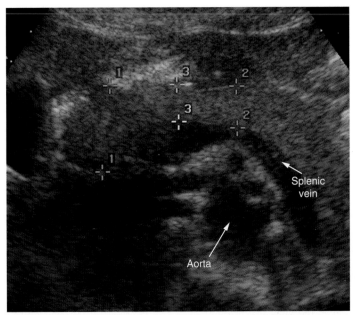

Figure 26 Axial plane through the pancreas at the level of the confluence of the splenic vein and superior mesenteric vein. Cursor 1 measures the anteroposterior depth of the pancreatic head, cursor 2 measures the anteroposterior diameter of the pancreatic body and cursor 3 measures the anteroposterior diameter of the pancreatic neck

REFERENCE
1. de Graaff CS, Taylor KJ, Simonds BD, Rosenfield AJ. Gray-scale echography of the pancreas. *Radiology* 1978;**129**:157–161.

FURTHER READING
Filly RA, London SS. The normal pancreas: acoustic characteristics and frequency of imaging. *Journal of Clinical Ultrasound* 1979;**7**:121–124.

Weill F, Schraub A, Eisenscher A, Bourgoin A. Ultrasonography of the normal pancreas. Success rate and criteria for normality. *Radiology* 1977;**123**:417–423.

Pancreatic duct (adult)

PREPARATION
None.

POSITION
Supine.

PROBE
2.0–5.0 MHz curvilinear transducer.

METHOD
The long axis of the pancreas should be determined. The duct in the region of the head–neck and body are obtained in the transverse/oblique planes. The diameter of the duct is taken as the distance between the inner layers of the anterior and posterior walls.

APPEARANCE
The duct appears as a low-reflective tubular structure with reflective walls. The lumen of the pancreatic duct is usually largest in the head of the pancreas and gradually decreases distally.

MEASUREMENTS

| | Normal pancreatic duct diameter (mm) | |
	Mean	Range
Head–neck	3.0	2.8–3.3
Proximal body	2.1	2.0–2.4
Distal body	1.6	1.0–1.7

The size of the pancreatic duct increases with age, with the upper limit of normal estimated at 3 mm. Administration of secretin causes pancreatic duct dilatation in normal subjects, but has no effect on dilatation caused by chronic pancreatitis and may be used to distinguish these two entities. The diameter of the pancreatic duct can increase during deep inspiration in adults without pancreatic disease; up to 1.3 mm when compared with images obtained at end-expiration.

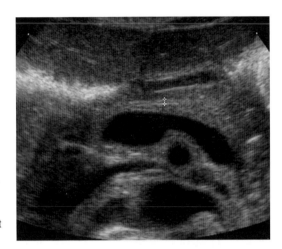

Figure 27 Axial plane through the pancreas, with cursors measuring the anteroposterior diameter of the pancreatic duct in the proximal aspect of the body

FURTHER READING

Glaser J, Hogemann B, Krummenerl T, Schneider M, Hultsch E, van Husen N, Gerlach U. Sonographic imaging of the pancreatic duct. New diagnostic possibilities using secretin stimulation. *Digestive Diseases and Sciences* 1987;**32**:1075–1081.

Hadidi A. Pancreatic duct diameter: sonographic measurement in normal subjects. *Journal of Clinical Ultrasound* 1983;**11**:17–22.

Wachsberg RH. Respiratory variation of the diameter of the pancreatic duct on sonography. *American Journal of Roentgenology* 2000;**175**:1459–1461.

Pancreas (pediatric)

PREPARATION
None.

POSITION
Supine, decubitus and semi-decubitus positions with the left side elevated.

PROBE
5.0–7.5 MHz curvilinear transducer.

METHOD
Maximum anteroposterior diameters of the head, body and tail of the pancreas are measured on transverse/oblique images.

APPEARANCE
The pancreas should be homogenous with a reflectivity equal to or slightly greater than that of adjacent liver. The pancreatic duct may be seen as a single high-reflective line and usually measures less than 1 mm.

MEASUREMENTS

Age	Anteroposterior dimensions of pancreas[1] (mean ± SD, cm)		
	Head	Body	Tail
<1 month	1.0 ± 0.4	0.6 ± 0.2	1.0 ± 0.4
1 month–1 year	1.5 ± 0.5	0.8 ± 0.3	1.2 ± 0.4
1–5 years	1.7 ± 0.3	1.0 ± 0.2	1.8 ± 0.4
5–10 years	1.6 ± 0.4	1.0 ± 0.3	1.8 ± 0.4
10–19 years	1.0 ± 0.5	1.1 ± 0.3	2.0 ± 0.4

Reproduced with permission from Siegel MJ, Martin KW, Worthington JL. Normal and abnormal pancreas in children. *Radiology* 1987;**165**:15–18.

REFERENCE

1. Siegel MJ, Martin KW, Worthington JL. Normal and abnormal pancreas in children. *Radiology* 1987;**165**:15–18.

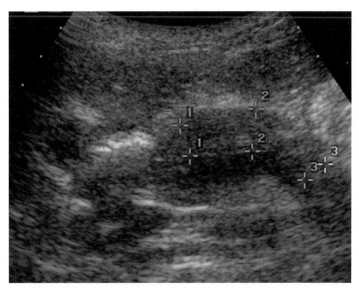

Figure 28   Axial plane through the pancreas at the level of the confluence of the splenic vein and superior mesenteric vein. Cursor 1 measures the anteroposterior depth of the pancreatic head, cursor 2 measures the anteroposterior diameter of the pancreatic body and cursor 3 measures the anteroposterior diameter of the pancreatic tail

Psoas muscle

PREPARATION
None.

POSITION
Supine.

PROBE
2.0–5.0 MHz curvilinear transducer.

METHOD
Longitudinal and transverse images from renal bed to iliac fossa.

APPEARANCE
Tubular low-reflective structure medial and posterior to the kidney. In longitudinal section may demonstrate high-reflective linear echoes, representing intramuscular tendon fibres. On a transverse section, a rounded low-reflective oval structure lateral to the spine is seen. In the iliac fossa psoas muscle blends with iliacus muscle. These appear as low-reflective soft tissue layers medial to curvilinear high reflectivity echo from distal shadowing of the iliac wing. A high-reflective region posterior and medial to the iliopsoas muscle represents the femoral nerve sheath. The psoas minor muscle cannot be identified as a separate structure.

FURTHER READING

King AD, Hine AL, McDonald C, Abrahams P. The ultrasound appearance of the normal psoas muscle. *Clinical Radiology* 1993;**48**:316–318.

Koenigsberg M, Hoffman JC, Schnur J. Sonographic evaluation of the retroperitoneum. *Seminars in Ultrasound* 1982;**3**:79–96.

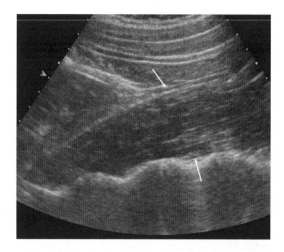

Figure 29a
Longitudinal plane through the lower pole of the right kidney demonstrating the linear high reflectivity of the intramuscular tendon fibers in the psoas muscle (between arrows)

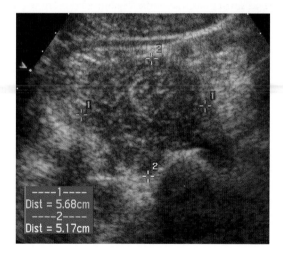

Figure 29b
Transverse section through the psoas muscle, again demonstrating the high-reflective tendon fibers

Retroperitoneal lymph nodes

PREPARATION
None.

POSITION
Supine.

PROBE
2.0–5.0 MHz curvilinear transducer.

METHOD
Longitudinal and transverse sections are used to image the aorta and the inferior vena cava. Lymphadenopathy is identified around these structures.

APPEARANCE
The appearances of normal lymph nodes are flattened, low-reflective structures with an eccentric highly reflective area representing the fatty hilum.

MEASUREMENT
It is frequently not possible to see normal sized glands of <1 cm. Lymph nodes greater than 1 cm are considered abnormally enlarged. Measurement is taken along the short axis.

FURTHER READING
Dietrich CF, Zeuzem S, Caspary WF, Wehrmann T. Ultrasound lymph node imaging in the abdomen and retroperitoneum of health probands. *Ultraschall in der Medizin* 1998;**19**:265–269.

Koenigsberg M, Hoffman JC, Schnur J. Sonographic evaluation of the retroperitoneum. *Seminars in Ultrasound* 1982;**3**:79–96.

Marchal G, Oyen R, Verschakelen J, Gelin J, Baert AL, Stessens RC. Sonographic appearance of normal lymph nodes. *Journal of Ultrasound in Medicine* 1985;**4**:417–419.

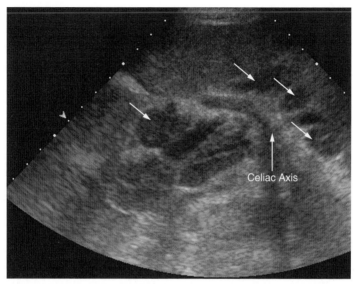

Figure 30 Oval low-reflective lymph nodes present (arrows) in the retroperitoneum around the celiac axis

4

ORGAN TRANSPLANTATION

Keshthra Satchithananda,
Zelena A. Aziz and
Paul S. Sidhu

Kidney transplantation	82
Renal artery stenosis in transplantation	86
Liver transplantation	88
Pancreas transplantation	92

Kidney transplantation

PREPARATION
None.

POSITION
Supine or right anterior oblique position.

PROBE
3.0–6.0 MHz curvilinear transducer.

METHOD
Renal transplants are normally situated in a retroperitoneal position in the right iliac fossa. The size may be measured in three planes, to calculate volume. Spectral Doppler waveforms from the upper, mid and lower aspects are obtained, aided by color Doppler imaging.

APPEARANCE
The transplant kidney may lie in various planes; there may be a prominent pelvicalyceal system. Corticomedullary differentiation may be readily visualized, and the renal sinus fat is of markedly high reflectivity.

MEASUREMENTS
- Volume = 0.51 × length × width × anteroposterior diameter

  If <90% of the immediate postoperative volume, consider chronic rejection or a vascular insult.

- The resistance index (RI) may be measured at the upper, mid and lower aspects of the transplant kidney, normally from an interlobular branch.

  RI = (peak systolic velocity – end diastolic velocity)/peak systolic velocity

The normal mean value is 0.64–0.73, abnormal if >0.75–0.90, but serial measurement changes over time are more important than single measurements.

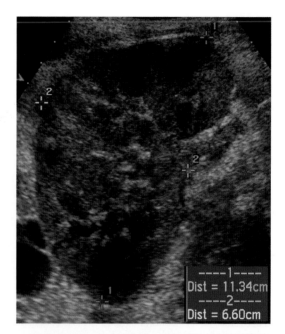

Figure 31a
Longitudinal plane
of a transplant
kidney in the right
iliac fossa

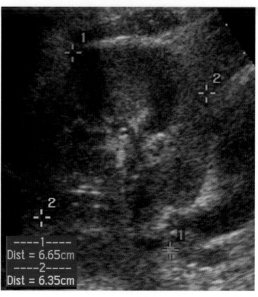

Figure 31b
Transverse plane of
the transplant
kidney. The size
may be measured
in three planes, to
calculate volume

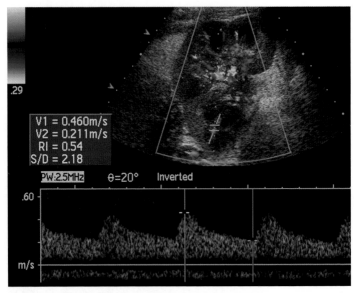

Figure 31c The resistance index is measured in this patient at the lower aspect of the transplant kidney, normally from an interlobular branch. (Courtesy of Dr. Colin R. Deane)

FURTHER READING

Absy M, Metreweli C, Matthews C, Al Khader A. Changes in transplanted kidney volume measured by ultrasound. *British Journal of Radiology* 1987;**60**:525–529.

Don S, Kopecky KK, Filo RS, Leapman SB, Thomalla JV, Jones JA, Klatte EC. Duplex Doppler US of renal allografts. Causes of elevated resistive index. *Radiology* 1989;**171**:709–712.

Hricak H, Lieto RP. Sonographic determination of renal volume. *Radiology* 1983;**148**:311–312.

Rifkin MD, Needleman L, Pasto ME, Kurtz AB, Foy PM, McGlynn E, Canino C, Baltarowich OH, Pennell RG, Goldberg BB. Evaluation of renal transplant rejection by duplex Doppler examination: value of resistive index. *American Journal of Roentgenology* 1987;**148**:759–762.

Renal artery stenosis in transplantation

PREPARATION
None.

POSITION
Supine or right anterior oblique position.

PROBE
3.0–6.0 MHz curvilinear transducer.

METHOD
Renal transplants are normally situated in a retroperitoneal position in the right iliac fossa. Doppler spectral analysis is performed along the length of the transplant artery, angle of insonation <60° using the lowest filter setting and a scale that accommodates the highest peak systolic velocities without aliasing.

APPEARANCE
- *Cadaver kidney:* harvested with an intact main renal artery and an attached portion of the aorta, sutured end-to-side of the recipient external iliac artery.
- *Living-related donor kidney:* main renal artery of the donor is sutured either directly end-to-side to the recipient external iliac artery or end-to-end to the recipient internal iliac artery.

MEASUREMENTS
- A peak systolic velocity (PSV) of ≤1.5 m/s is usually considered normal. A transplant renal artery with a PSV ≥2.0 m/s is suggestive of a >50% diameter reduction.
- Ratio of PSV in the transplant renal artery to the PSV in the external iliac artery. There is considerable variation in the PSV of the transplant artery, and a ratio can be used; the upper limit should not exceed 1.5.
- Changes in the resistance index (RI), acceleration index (gradient of the systolic upstroke) and acceleration time (time taken from the beginning of the systolic upstroke to the first systolic peak) recorded in the intrarenal vessels are less useful as a discrimatory diagnostic test.

  RI = (peak systolic velocity – end diastolic velocity)/peak systolic velocity

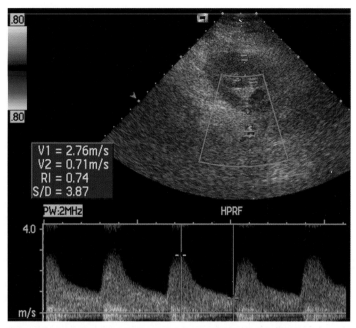

Figure 32 A transplant renal artery with a peak systolic velocity of 2.76 m/s is suggestive of a >50% diameter reduction (Courtesy of Dr. Colin R. Deane)

FURTHER READING

Baxter GM, Ireland H, Moss JG, Harden PN, Junor BJR, Rodger RSC. Colour Doppler ultrasound in renal transplant artery stenosis; which Doppler index? *Clinical Radiology* 1995;**50**:618–622.

Cochlin DLL, Wake A, Salaman JR, Griffin PJA. Ultrasound changes in the transplant kidney. *Clinical Radiology* 1988;**39**:373–376.

Dodd GD, Tublin ME, Shah A, Zajko AB. Imaging of vascular complications associated with renal transplants. *American Journal of Roentgenology* 1991;**157**:449–459.

Liver transplantation

PREPARATION
None.

POSITION
Supine or right anterior oblique position.

PROBE
3.0–5.0 MHz curvilinear transducer.

METHOD
Ultrasound is the primary screening technique for detection of vascular complications of hepatic transplantation. Longitudinal and transverse images are taken from a subcostal or intercostal approach on inspiration in the supine and right anterior oblique positions.

APPEARANCE
Liver parenchyma should be of uniform medium strength echoes.

- *Hepatic artery:* Visualized at the porta hepatis. Normal hepatic artery Doppler waveform shows a low-resistance flow pattern with continuous diastolic flow. Complications are hepatic artery thrombosis, manifest as absence of hepatic artery and intrahepatic arterial flow. Sometimes flow is detected in the intrahepatic location due to collateral vessel formation. A tardus parvus waveform is a characteristic change in arterial flow distal to a stenosis. Absence of arterial flow at the porta hepatis with tardus parvus waveform distally within an intrahepatic artery is suggestive of main artery thrombosis

- *Portal vein:* Visualized at the porta hepatis. Normal portal vein Doppler waveform shows continuous flow pattern with mild velocity variations induced by respiration. Complications include portal vein thrombosis and stenosis. Thrombosis is seen on grayscale ultrasound as high-reflective luminal thrombus or narrowing. Color and spectral Doppler ultrasound shows no detectable flow in the portal vein.

- *Hepatic veins and inferior vena cava (IVC):* Doppler spectral waveforms of the hepatic veins and IVC are similar with phasic flow pattern indicative of physiologic changes in blood flow with cardiac cycle.

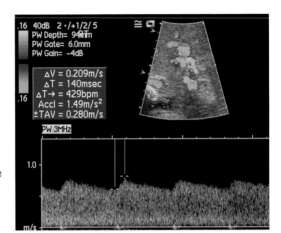

Figure 33a A spectral Doppler gate is placed over the intrahepatic hepatic artery and an acceleration time of 140 ms is measured, indicating a 'tardus parvus' waveform

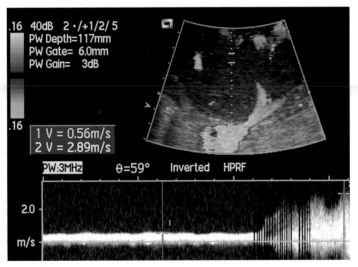

Figure 33b A spectral Doppler gate is placed over the distal hepatic vein at the anastomosis with the suprahepatic inferior vena cava and an increase in velocity from 0.56 m/s to 2.89 m/s indicates a focal stenosis in the hepatic vein

MEASUREMENTS

- A tardus parvus waveform is a characteristic change in arterial flow distal to a stenosis. This waveform has a resistance index (RI) <0.5 and a systolic acceleration time (time from end diastole to first systolic peak) >0.12 s.
- Stenosis of portal vein shows focal color aliasing with a >3–4 fold increase in velocity relative to the prestenotic segment, or an absolute velocity measurement of >100 cm/s at the site of the stenosis.
- Thrombosis or stenosis of IVC can occur after transplantation and the latter is usually at the site of the anastomosis. Grayscale ultrasound shows high-reflective thrombus or obvious narrowing. Spectral Doppler evaluation shows a 3-4-fold increase in velocity across the stenosis with loss of normal caval phasicity in the hepatic venous spectral Doppler waveform. Loss of phasicity in the hepatic veins also indicates upper caval anastomotic stenosis.

FURTHER READING

Nghiem HV, Tran K, Winter III TC, Schmidt UP, Althaus SJ, Patel NH, Freeny PC. Imaging of complications of liver transplantation. *Radiographics* 1996;**16**:825–840.

Ryan SM, Sidhu PS. Early post-operative liver transplant ultrasound. In: Sidhu PS, Baxter GM. eds. *Ultrasound of abdominal transplantation*. Thieme, Stuttgart, 2002, pp. 90–104.

Shaw AS, Ryan SM, Beese RC, Norris S, Bowles M, Rela M, Sidhu PS. Liver transplantation. *Imaging* 2002; **14**:314–328.

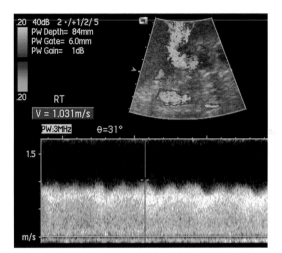

Figure 33c A spectral Doppler gate is placed over the intrahepatic portal vein, and an absolute velocity measurement of 1.03 m/s is obtained, indicating the presence of portal vein stenosis

Pancreas transplantation

PREPARATION
None.

POSITION
Supine or right anterior oblique position.

PROBE
3.0–5.0 MHz curvilinear transducer.

METHOD
Commonly the entire pancreas is transplanted with a section of duodenum anastomosed to the bladder. The gland is situated in the pelvis, with the venous anastomosis between the donor portal vein and the anterior aspect of the recipient external or common iliac vein. The arterial anastomosis is from the recipient anterior wall of the common iliac artery to a patch of donor aorta containing the celiac trunk and superior mesenteric artery.

APPEARANCE
Uniform pattern of reflectivity similar to that of muscle. Rejection appears as gland enlargement, focal or diffuse areas of low reflectivity, and a resistance index (RI) of >0.7 (measured in the donor arterial trunk). Imaging is paramount in follow up of pancreatic transplant as clinical and biochemical evaluation is relatively insensitive in determining episodes of acute rejection. Ultrasound evaluation and guidance will allow percutaneous biopsy to confirm the diagnosis and institute therapy. Pancreatic duct exocrine drainage is via the bladder.

MEASUREMENTS
- Anteroposterior size of normal gland: head 3 cm, body 2.5 cm, tail 2.5 cm. Pancreatic duct should be ≤3 mm.
- Color Doppler to locate and show patency of main graft artery and vein.
- RI of the artery should be ≤0.7.

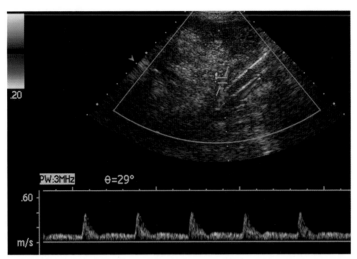

Figure 34 Color Doppler to locate and show patency of main graft artery and vein. A spectral Doppler gate records the spectral waveform from which the resistance index is calculated (Courtesy of Dr. Colin R. Deane)

FURTHER READING

Green SJ, Sidhu PS, Deane CR. Imaging of simultaneous kidney pancreatic transplants. *Imaging* 2002; **14**:299–307.

Patel B, Wolverson MK, Mahanta B. Pancreatic transplant rejection: assessment with duplex US. *Radiology* 1989;**173**:131–135.

Wong JJ, Krebs TL, Klassen DK, Daly B, Simon EM, Bartlett ST, Grumbach K, Drachenberg CB. Sonographic evaluation of acute pancreatic transplant rejection: Morphology–Doppler analysis versus guided percutaneous biopsy. *American Journal of Roentgenology* 1996;**166**:803–807.

Yuh WT, Wise JA, Abu-Yousef MM, Rezai K, Sato Y, Berbaum KS, Kao SC, Hunsicker LG, Corry RJ. Pancreatic transplant imaging. *Radiology* 1988;**167**:679–683.

5 PELVIS

Bladder   96
   Bladder volume and residual
     volume   96
   Bladder wall   100
   Ureterovesical jets (pediatric and
     infant)   102
Male genital tract   104
   Testes   104
   Epididymis   108
   Prostate – transrectal sonography   110
   Seminal vesicles – transrectal
     sonography   112
   Penis   114
Female urogenital tract   118
   Ovary – transvaginal sonography   118
   Ovarian follicles – transvaginal
     sonography   120
   Cervix – transvaginal sonography   122
   Uterus – transvaginal sonography   124
   Endometrial stripe – transvaginal
     sonography   126
   Urethra   128
   Length of the cervix and cervical
     canal in pregnancy   130

BLADDER

Keshthra Satchithananda,
Zelena A. Aziz and
Paul S. Sidhu

Bladder volume and residual volume

PREPARATION
Full bladder is required

POSITION
Supine.

PROBE
3.0–5.0 MHz curvilinear transducer.

METHOD
Transverse plane for the width and depth, and then a longitudinal image provides the length and depth measurements. Measurements are estimated both before and after micturition. There should be no post-micturition residual volume.

APPEARANCE
When full, the bladder is clearly defined as an almost square structure of low reflectivity in the transverse plane. Within the bladder the trigone is the area containing the ureteric and urethral orifices. The urethral orifice marks the bladder neck.

MEASUREMENTS

blood volume (ml) = $(\pi/6) \times$ length $\times$ depth $\times$ width

($\pi/6$ may be substituted by 0.51)

The accuracy of this calculation is variable, as it is based on an ellipsoid formula, and there is considerable variation in bladder shape. At least 200 ml of fluid must be in the bladder to make a urodynamic flow rate study accurate. If there remains a >100 ml residual volume, the patient should attempt further bladder emptying and the examination repeated.

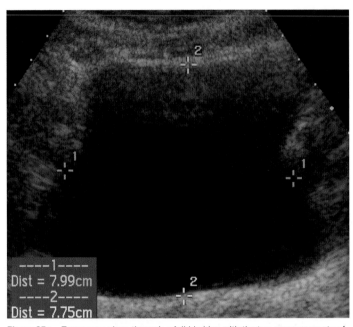

Figure 35a Transverse plane through a full bladder, with the two measurements of width and depth obtained

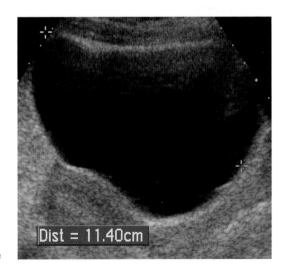

Figure 35b Longitudinal plane with the measurement of length obtained in order to calculate the bladder volume

FURTHER READING

McLean GK, Edell SL. Determination of bladder volumes by gray scale ultrasonography. *Radiology* 1978;**128**:181–182.

Griffiths CJ, Murray A, Ramsden PD. Accuracy and repeatability of bladder volume measurement using ultrasonic imaging. *Journal of Urology* 1986;**136**:808–812.

Poston GJ, Joseph AE, Riddle PR. The accuracy of ultrasound in the measurement of changes in bladder volume. *British Journal of Urology* 1983;**55**:361–363.

Bladder wall

PREPARATION
Full bladder is required

POSITION
Supine.

PROBE
3.0–5.0 MHz curvilinear transducer.

METHOD
Bladder wall is measured on transverse and longitudinal images by placing the probe in the midline above the pubis. On transverse views the bladder floor lateral to the trigone and on longitudinal views the posterior inferior wall are the optimal sites for measurement.

APPEARANCE
Smooth contour with the high-reflective mucosa distinguishable from the low-reflective detrusor muscle.

MEASUREMENTS
Regardless of the patient's age and gender:
- normal empty bladder ≤5 mm
- well-distended bladder ≤3 mm

FURTHER READING

Jequier S, Rousseau O. Sonographic measurements of the normal bladder wall in children. *American Journal of Roentgenology* 1987;**149**:563–566.

Manieri C, Carter SSC, Romano G, Trucchi A, Valenti M, Tubaro A. The diagnosis of bladder outlet obstruction in men by ultrasound measurement of bladder wall thickness. *Journal of Urology* 1998;**159**:761–765.

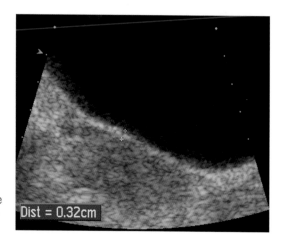

Figure 36
Longitudinal plane, measuring the depth of the posterior wall of the bladder adjacent to the uterus

Ureterovesical jets (pediatric and infant)

PREPARATION
Ingestion of water

POSITION
Supine.

PROBE
5.0–7.5 MHz curvilinear transducer.

METHOD
Transverse image through the bladder base. The site of the ureteric orifice is usually lateral and defined as the ureteovesical junction at the apex of the angle between the bladder floor and the lateral wall, or in the lateral vertical wall of the bladder, above the bladder floor.

APPEARANCE
The ureteric jet is seen on grayscale when there is a difference of at least 0.01 g/ml between the specific gravity of urine coming down the ureter and the urine present in the bladder. When a spectral Doppler gate is placed onto the jet, a characteristic signal is obtained even when the jet is not seen on grayscale. Color Doppler flow imaging is more sensitive in demonstrating flow than grayscale and facilitates location of the ureteric orifice.

MEASUREMENTS
In children with normal voiding cystourethrogram (VCUG) and normal renal and bladder ultrasound:
- Duration of jet: right, 2.77 ± 1.5 s, and left 2.88 ± 1.5 s
- Direction of jet: Usually anteromedial and upward
- Spectral analysis: 10–80 cm/s (mean of 31.6 cm/s)

Frequency of jets and resultant signal increase with urine production; an almost continuous signal is obtained after a large fluid load. Although identification of ureterovesical jets may be made on ultrasound, there are no specific features regarding the jets that reliably distinguish a normal from an abnormal ureterovesical junction.

FURTHER READING
Jequier S, Paltiel H, Lafortune M. Uretero-vesical jets in infants and children: duplex and color Doppler studies. *Radiology* 1990;**175**:349–353.

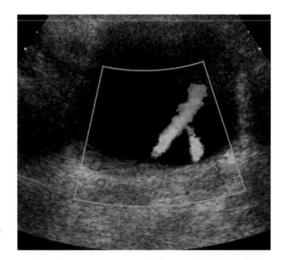

Figure 37a Color Doppler image of the right and left ureteric jets demonstrating the anteromedial and upward direction of the jet

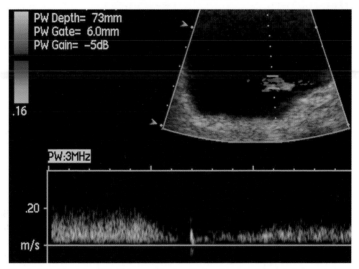

Figure 37b A spectral Doppler gate is placed over the ureteric jet, and a spectral waveform obtained (Courtesy of Meena Shah)

MALE GENITAL TRACT

Zelena A. Aziz,
Keshthra Satchithananda and
Paul S. Sidhu

Testes

PREPARATION
None.

POSITION
Supine, with towel beneath the scrotum to provide support.

PROBE
7.0–13.0 MHz linear transducer.

METHOD
Compare reflectivity between the two sides on a single image. Obtain transverse and longitudinal images.

APPEARANCE
The testes are homogenous and of medium-level reflectivity. The mediastinum testis is a highly reflective linear structure in the posterior–superior aspect of the testicle draining the seminiferous tubules of the testes into the rete testis. Drainage from here is via the epididymis to the seminal vesicles. The rete testis is a low-reflective area at the hilum of the testis with finger-like projections into the parenchyma. Apart from these projections, the parenchyma of the testis should remain of homogenous reflectivity. The appendix testis (a vestigial remnant of the müllerian duct) is present in the majority of patients, most commonly at the superior testicular pole or in the groove between the testis and the head of the epididymis medially. There is marked variation in its size and appearance; it is usually oval, although a stalk-like structure is occasionally seen.

MEASUREMENTS
- Average size is $3.8 \times 3.0 \times 2.5$ cm. The length can be up to 5 cm.
- Volume measurement is calculated using the formula:

  length $\times$ width $\times$ height $\times 0.51$.

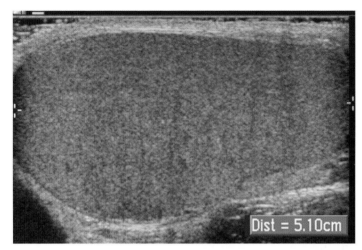

Figure 38a Longitudinal plane through the testis demonstrating homogenous medium-level reflectivity

Figure 38b
Transverse section through the same testis. Volume can be calculated from the three measurements obtained

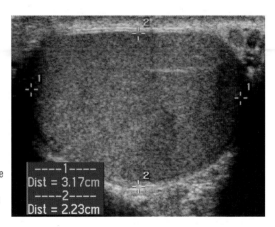

- A total volume (both testes) of >30 ml is indicative of normal function. Testicular volume >2 ml allows reliable appreciation of intra-testicular color Doppler flow. A varicocele is present if the vein measures > 2 mm.

FURTHER READING

Ingram S, Hollman AS. Colour Doppler sonography of the normal paediatric testis. *Clinical Radiology* 1994;**49**:266–267.

Leung ML, Gooding GAW, Williams RD. High-resolution sonography of scrotal contents in asymptomatic subjects. *American Journal of Roentgenology* 1984;**143**:161–164.

Paltiel HJ, Diamond DA, Di Canzio J, Zurakowski D, Borer JG, Atala A. Testicular volume: comparison of orchidometer and US measurements in dogs. *Radiology* 2002;**222**:114–119.

Sellars MEK, Sidhu PS. Pictorial review: Ultrasound imaging of the rete testis. *European Journal of Ultrasound* 2001;**14**:115–120.

Sellars MEK, Sidhu PS. Ultrasound appearances of the testicular appendages: pictorial review. *European Radiology* 2003;**13**:127–135.

Epididymis

PREPARATION
None.

POSITION
Supine, with towel beneath the scrotum to provide support.

PROBE
7.0–10.0 MHz linear transducer.

METHOD
Transverse and longitudinal images, to include the head, body and tail.

APPEARANCE
The epididymis is 6–7 cm in length. The head (globus major) is a pyramid-shaped structure lying superior to the upper pole of the testis. The body courses along the posterolateral aspect of the testicle. The tail (globus minor) is slightly thicker than the body and can be seen as a curved structure at the inferior aspect of the testicle where it becomes the proximal portion of the ductus deferens. The body and tail are of similar or slightly lower reflectivity than the testis; the head is of slightly higher reflectivity. The appendix epididymis is not as frequently seen as the appendix testis. It is part of the mesonephric (wolffian duct), and projects from the epididymis from different sites, most commonly the head. It usually has a stalk-like appearance.

MEASUREMENTS
The globus major measures 10–12 mm in diameter, the body less than 4 mm (average 1–2 mm) in diameter.

FURTHER READING
Krone KD, Carroll BA. Scrotal ultrasound. *Radiologic Clinics of North America* 1985;**23**:121–139.

Leung ML, Gooding GAW, Williams RD. High-resolution sonography of scrotal contents in asymptomatic subjects. *American Journal of Roentgenology* 1984;**143**:161–164.

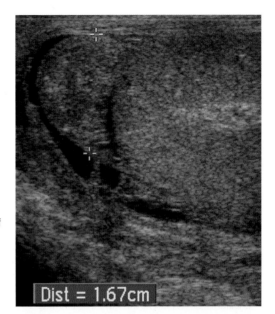

Figure 39a A longitudinal plane through the head of the epididymis in a patient with acute epididymitis with the depth of the epididymal head measuring 1.67 cm

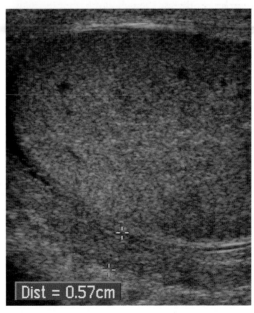

Figure 39b The body of the epididymis in the same patient measuring 0.57 cm

Prostate – transrectal sonography

PREPARATION
None.

POSITION
Left lateral.

PROBE
A dedicated transrectal probe is used which may vary in frequency from 5.0–7.5 MHz. Single or multi-plane probes may be used.

METHOD
The examination is best performed with the patient's bladder half full to provide a contrast to the high-reflective perivesicular fat surrounding the prostate. Axial and longitudinal images can be obtained.

APPEARANCE
The prostate is usefully separated into a peripheral zone and an inner gland (encompassing the transition and central zones, and periurethral glandular area). The peripheral zone encompasses 70% of the glandular tissue, appears as medium-level uniform low reflectivity, separated from the central zone by the surgical capsule, which is often of high reflectivity.

MEASUREMENTS
Measurement of anteroposterior (H), transverse (W) and cephalo-caudal (L) dimensions, with the volume calculated using the formula:

$\pi/6 \times H \times W \times L$ ($\pi/6$ may be substituted by 0.51)

The normal prostate measures 2.5–3.0 × 2.5–3.0 × 2.0–2.5 cm, with an estimated volume of 20 ml.

FURTHER READING
Terris MK, Stamey TA. Determination of prostate volume by transrectal ultrasound. *Journal of Urology* 1991;**145**:984–987.
Villers A, Terris MK, McNeal JE, Stamey TA. Ultrasound anatomy of the prostate: the normal gland and anatomical variations. *Journal of Urology* 1990;**143**:732–738.

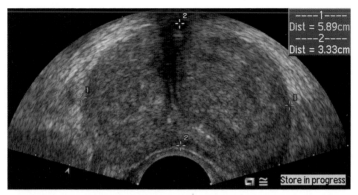

Figure 40a Anteroposterior and transverse measurements of an enlarged prostate

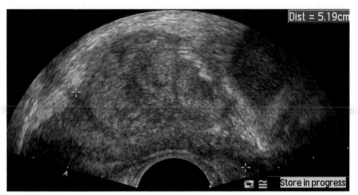

Figure 40b Cephalocaudal measurements in the same patient (Courtesy of Dr. Ian Stanton)

Seminal vesicles – transrectal sonography

PREPARATION
None.

POSITION
Left lateral.

PROBE
A dedicated transrectal probe is used which may vary in frequency from 5.0–7.5 MHz. Single or multi-plane probes may be used.

METHOD
The examination is best performed with the patient's bladder half full to provide a contrast to the high-reflective perivesicular fat surrounding the seminal vesicles. Axial and longitudinal images can be obtained.

APPEARANCE
The seminal vesicles are seen as flat, paired structures lying behind the bladder. The centre of the gland is of low reflectivity, with areas of high reflectivity corresponding to the folds of the excretory epithelium. If distended, the wall can be seen to be composed of two layers. The vas deferens bilaterally can be identified behind the bladder as they run inward and posteriorly to become the ampulla. The junction of the seminal vesicle with the ejaculatory duct usually lies well within the prostate. The ejaculatory complex from each side lies in a communal muscular envelope, which can be identified; the actual lumen of the normal ejaculatory ducts is not normally visible.

MEASUREMENTS
Measurement of anteroposterior, transverse and cephalocaudal dimensions, with the volume calculated using the formula:

volume (ml) = (anteroposterior dimension × transverse dimension × cephalocaudal dimension)/2

Age (years)	Bilateral volume[1] (mean $\pm$ SD, ml)
20–29	9.3 ± 3.9
30–39	9.7 ± 1.3
40–49	10.1 ± 2.6
50–59	9.3 ± 2.4
60–69	7.5 ± 1.7
70–79	6.1 ± 4.5
80–89	5.1 ± 1.1

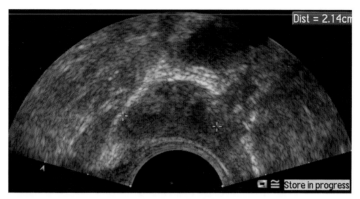

Figure 41a Cephalocaudal measurements of the seminal vesicles

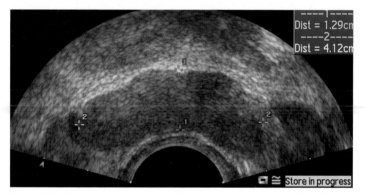

Figure 41b Anteroposterior and transverse measurements of the seminal vesicles in the same patient (Courtesy of Dr. Ian Stanton)

FURTHER READING

Carter SSC, Shinohara K, Lipshultz LI. Transrectal ultrasonography in disorders of the seminal vesicles and ejaculatory ducts. *Urologic Clinics of North America* 1989;**16**:773–789.

REFERENCE

1. Terasaki T, Watanabe H, Kamoi K, Naya Y. Seminal vesicle parameters at 10-year intervals measured by transrectal ultrasonography. *Journal of Urology* 1993;**150**:914–916.

Penis

PREPARATION
None.

POSITION
Patient is supine, and the penis is examined on the dorsal aspect.

PROBE
7.5–10.0 MHz linear transducer.

APPEARANCE
The body of the penis consists of two corpora cavernosa and the corpus spongiosum (containing the urethra), which lies on the ventral surface of the fused corpora cavernosa. The cavernosal artery and the dorsal artery supply the penis. Pharmaco-stimulation with color and spectral Doppler ultrasound allows for the assessment of arterial flow disorders as well as of venous leakage in erectile dysfunction.

METHOD
The penis is imaged longitudinally and transversely in the flaccid state to detect areas of fibrosis and calcification to indicate Peyronie's disease. A baseline assessment of the spectral Doppler waveform of the right cavernosal artery, as close to the base of the penis as possible, is made, recording the peak systolic velocity (PSV) in a longitudinal plane, and with a Doppler angle of <60°. Following the intracavernosal injection of 20 µg prostaglandin E_1 (PGE1), measurements of the PSV and end-diastolic velocity (EDV) are made every 5 minutes for 20 minutes at the same level in the right cavernosal artery.

MEASUREMENTS
A guide to differentiation among arteriogenic, venogenic and nonvascular dysfunction assessed 15 minutes after cavernous stimulation with 20 µg PGE1. Without adequate arterial input, measurements of the EDV are of limited value.

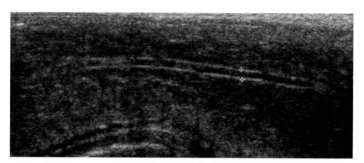

Figure 42a Longitudinal image through the penis with the cursors indicating a dilated cavernosal artery following pharmacostimulation

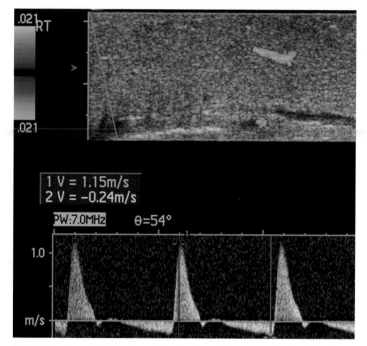

Figure 42b A spectral Doppler gate is placed over the cavernosal artery 20 minutes after pharmacostimulation with a spectral Doppler waveform indicating a normal response. The peak systolic velocity is 1.15 m/s and there is reversal of flow in diastole

Type of dysfunction	PSV (cm/s)	EDV (cm/s)
Arteriogenic	<25	<5
Venogenic	>25	>5
Normal values	>30	<5

FURTHER READING

Andresen R, Wegner HEH. Assessment of the penile vascular system with color-coded duplex sonography and pharmacocavernosometry and -graphy in impotent men. *Acta Radiologica* 1997;**38**:303–308.

Benson CB, Aruny JE, Vickers MA. Correlation of duplex sonography with arteriography in patients with erectile dysfunction. *American Journal of Roentgenology* 1993;**160**:71–73.

Quam JP, King BF, James EM, Lewis RW, Brakke DM, Ilstrup DM, Parulkar BG, Hattery RR. Duplex and color sonographic evaluation of vasculogenic impotence. *American Journal of Roentgenology* 1989;**153**:1141–1147.

FEMALE UROGENITAL TRACT

Kelley Z. Allison and
Wui K. Chong

Ovary – transvaginal sonography

PREPARATION
Empty bladder before examination.

POSITION
Lithotomy position on adapted examination couch.

PROBE
8.4 MHz curved transvaginal transducer.

METHOD
The longest diameter of the ovaries is obtained (d1). The maximum anteroposterior diameter (d2) is obtained perpendicular to d1. The transducer is then rotated 90° and d3 is measured perpendicular to d2.

APPEARANCE
Ovoid structure between uterus and muscular pelvic sidewall. The internal iliac vessels are posterior to the ovaries. The presence of follicles is the hallmark in their identification.

MEASUREMENT

ovarian volume = d1 × d2 × d3 × 0.523

Category	Age	Average volume (mean ± SD, ml)
Pediatric	2–14 years	1.0–4.1 ± 3.0
Adult	Premenopausal	4.9 ± 0.03 (upper limit 20)
	Postmenopausal	2.2 ± 0.01 (upper limit 10)

FURTHER READING
Pavlik EJ, DePriest PD, Gallion HH, Ueland FR, Reedy MB, Kryscio RJ, van Nagell JR Jr. Ovarian volume related to age. *Gynaecologic Oncology* 2001;80:333–334.

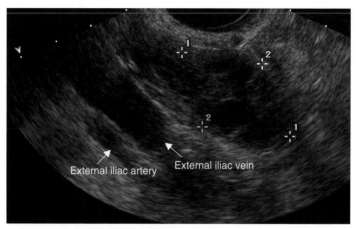

Figure 43 Ovoid structure between uterus and muscular pelvic sidewall, with the internal iliac vessels posterior (Courtesy of Sue Rzepka)

Ovarian follicles – transvaginal sonography

PREPARATION
Empty bladder before examination.

POSITION
Lithotomy position on adapted examination couch.

PROBE
8.4 MHz curved transvaginal transducer.

METHOD
Maximum diameter of follicle is obtained.

APPEARANCE
The ovary is the ovoid structure between uterus and muscular pelvic sidewall. The internal iliac vessels are posterior to the ovaries. Follicles are seen as echo-free ovoid structures within the ovary.

MEASUREMENT
Number of follicles: ≤5 follicles per ovary.

Category	Size
Dominant follicle	20–27 mm
(day prior to ovulation)	<25 mm
Non-dominant follicle	<14 mm
Hormone treatment	Same size but more than one dominant follicle (3–5)

FURTHER READING
Pache TD, Wladimiroff JW, Hop WC, Fauser BC. How to discriminate between normal and polycystic ovaries: transvaginal US study. *Radiology* 1992;**183**:421–423.

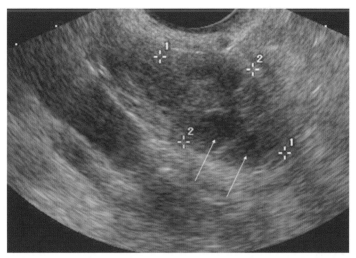

Figure 44 The presence of follicles (arrows) seen as low-reflective ovoid structures within the ovary, with the diameter measured as the maximum diameter (Courtesy of Sue Rzepka)

Cervix – transvaginal sonography

PREPARATION
Empty bladder before examination.

POSITION
Lithotomy position on adapted examination couch.

PROBE
8.4 MHz curved transvaginal transducer.

METHOD
Sagittal image of cervix is obtained with the probe in the anterior fornix. The cervix is measured linearly between the external os at its junction with the vaginal mucosa inferiorly and the internal os at the point where it widens into the lower uterine segment. The translabial (transperineal) cervical length demonstrates close correlation with the transvaginal measurement.

APPEARANCE
The cervix is fixed in the midline, of midlevel echogenicity. The endocervical canal appears as a high-reflective line, surrounded by a low-reflective zone (endocervical glands). In the gravid patient, the lower uterine segment and the cervix have a Y-shaped configuration.

MEASUREMENT

Age	Average length (range, cm)
Premenopausal	2.3–3.6
Postmenopausal	2.1–2.6

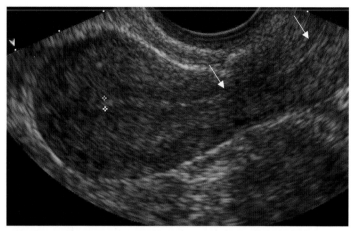

Figure 45   The cervix is measured from the cervical tip inferiorly to the point of widening of lower uterine segment (arrows) (Courtesy of Sue Rzepka)

FURTHER READING

Baltarowich OH. Female pelvic organ measurements. In Goldberg BB, Keertz AB (eds) *Atlas of Ultrasound Measurements*, 1990. Chicago: Year Book Medical Publishers.

Kurtzman JT, Goldsmith LJ, Gall SA, Spinnato JA. Transvaginal versus transperineal ultrasonography: a blinded comparison in the assessment of cervical length at midgestation. *American Journal of Obstetrics and Gynecology* 1998;**179**:852–857.

Uterus – transvaginal sonography

PREPARATION
Empty bladder before examination.

POSITION
Lithotomy position on adapted examination couch.

PROBE
8.4 MHz curved transvaginal transducer.

METHOD
The transducer is oriented in a longitudinal plane of the uterus and the midline position is confirmed by the endocervical/endometrial cavity. The total uterine length is measured from the top of the fundus to the external cervical os. The maximum anteroposterior (AP) diameter is measured perpendicular to the maximum length. The transducer is the rotated 90° at the level of AP to obtain maximum transverse (TRV) diameter.

APPEARANCE
Uniform pattern of medium strength echos with a high-reflective central stripe (endometrial stripe).

MEASUREMENT

Age	Dimensions (mean ± SD, cm)		
	Length	AP	TRV
Prepubertal			
(8–13 years)	3.6–5.4 ± 1.1	0.9–1.6 ± 0.4	1.8–2.9 (range)
Premenopausal			
Nulliparous	7.1 ± 0.8	3.3 ± 0.08	4.6 ± 0.6
Parous	8.9 ± 1.0	4.3 ± 0.6	5.8 ± 0.8
Postmenopausal	7.9 ± 1.2	3.2 ± 0.7	4.9 ± 0.8

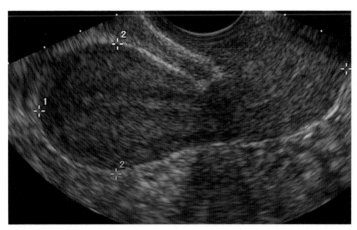

Figure 46 The total uterine length (cursors 1) measured from the fundus to the external cervical os. The maximum anteroposterior (cursors 2) diameter is measured perpendicular to the maximum length (Courtesy of Sue Rzepka)

FURTHER READING

Miller EI, Thomas RH, Lines P. The atrophic postmenopausal uterus. *Journal of Clinical Ultrasound* 1977;**5**:261–263.

Platt JF, Bree RL, Davidson D. Ultrasound of the normal non-gravid uterus: correlation with gross and histopathology. *Journal of Clinical Ultrasound* 1990;**18**:15–19.

Siegel MJ. Pediatric gynecologic sonography. *Radiology* 1991;**179**:593–600.

Endometrial stripe – transvaginal sonography

PREPARATION
Empty bladder before examination.

POSITION
Lithotomy position on adapted examination couch.

PROBE
8.4 MHz curved transvaginal transducer.

METHOD
Midline sagittal view of uterus. Measure the outer edge to outer edge of high-reflective interfaces.

APPEARANCE
- *Proliferative phase:* Thin high-reflective line representing endometrial cavity interface, low-reflective superficial layer and high-reflective deep layer.
- *Secretory phase:* Homogenously high-reflective stripe surrounded by low-reflective zone representing the hypervascular portion of myometrium.

MEASUREMENT

Age group	Phase of cycle	Thickness (mm)
Premenopausal	Menstrual	2–3
	Early proliferative	4–6
	Periovulatory	6–8
	Secretory	8–15
Postmenopausal		
	Hormone replacement	≤8
	Not on hormone	≤5

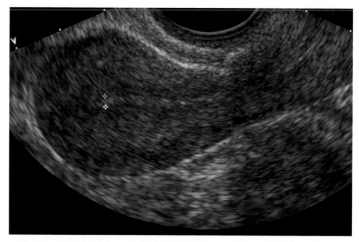

Figure 47 Midline sagittal view of uterus, with a measure from the outer edge to outer edge of high-reflective interfaces (Courtesy of Sue Rzepka)

FURTHER READING

Borstein J, Auslender R, Goldstein S, Kohan R, Stolar Z, Abramovici H. Increased endometrial thickness in women with hypertension. *American Journal of Obstetrics and Gynecology* 2000;**183**:583–587.

Brooks SE, Yeatts-Peterson M, Baker SP, Reuter KL. Thickened endometrial stripe and/or endometrial fluid as a marker of pathology: fact or fancy? *Gynecologic Oncology* 1996;**63**:19–24.

Urethra

PREPARATION
A full bladder is required.

POSITION
Supine.

PROBE
3.5–5.0 MHz curvilinear transducer.

METHOD
Images of the urethra can be acquired in the transverse and sagittal planes.

APPEARANCE
The urethra consists of muscular, erectile and mucous layers with a central lumen. This gives an ovoid 'bull's eye' appearance on transverse scans. The reflectivity is similar to that of vaginal tissues; both are of lower reflectivity than the surrounding connective tissue or the bladder wall.

MEASUREMENTS
The anteroposterior diameter of the female urethra, just inferior to the bladder, measures 1–1.5 cm.

FURTHER READING
Hennigan HW Jr, Dubose TJ. Sonography of the female urethra.
American Journal of Roentgenology 1985;**145**:839–841.

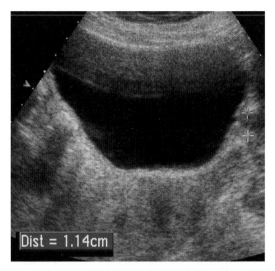

Figure 48a
Longitudinal image demonstrating the urethra (between cursors), which has a reflectivity similar to that of vaginal tissues, lower reflectivity than the surrounding connective tissue or the bladder wall

Dist = 1.14cm

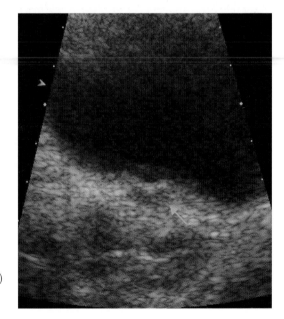

Figure 48b
Transverse image demonstrating the 'bull-eyes' appearance (arrow) (Courtesy of Olivia Benson-Fadayomi)

Length of the cervix and cervical canal in pregnancy

PREPARATION
Partially distended bladder for transabdominal imaging in the second trimester. Avoid overdistension of bladder, which artificially increases cervical length.

POSITION
Sagittal image of uterus and cervix

PROBE
- Transabdominal or translabial 3–5 MHz curvilinear transducer
- Transvaginal 5–8.0 MHz transducer

METHOD
Length of cervical canal from internal to external os. this can be measured transabdominally, transvaginally or translabially.

APPEARANCE
Cylindrical structure with echogenic central canal. The internal os is the junction of the amniotic sac and the cervical canal. The external os is the lower end of the cervical canal, where the anterior and posterior lips of the cervix meet.

MEASUREMENTS

Approach	Length (mm)
Transvaginal	32–48
Translabial	29–35
Transabdominal	
(maternal bladder partially or fully distended)	32–53
Empty[1]	32.5

Cervical length of <20 mm on transvaginal sonography is suggestive of cervical incompetence.[2,3]

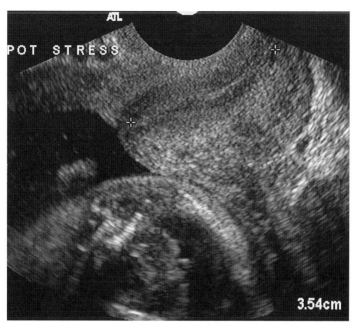

Figure 49 The distance from the internal os (junction of the amniotic sac and the cervical canal) to the external os (lower end of the cervical canal) is measured (cursors) (Courtesy of Anthony E. Swartz)

REFERENCES

1. Bowie JD, Andreotti RF, Rosenberg ER. Sonographic appearance of the uterine cervix in pregnancy: the vertical cervix. *American Journal of Roentgenology* 1983;**140**:737–740.
2. Iams JD, Goldenberg RL, Meis PJ, Mercer BM, Moawad A, Das A, Thom E, McNellis D, Copper RL, Johnson F, Roberts JM. The length of the cervix and the risk of spontaneous premature delivery. New England Journal of Medicine 1996;**334**:567–572.
3. Guzman ER, Mellon C, Vintzileos AM, Ananth CV, Walteis C, Gipson, K. Longitudinal assessment of endocervical length between 15 and 24 weeks gestation in women at risk for pregnancy loss or preterm birth. *Obstetrics Gynecology* 1998;**92**:31–37.

6 SUPERFICIAL STRUCTURES

Keshthra Satchithananda,
Zelena A. Aziz and
Paul S. Sidhu

Parathyroid glands	134
Submandibular salivary glands	136
Parotid salivary glands	138
Thyroid gland	140
Lymph nodes in the neck	144
Orbits – extraocular muscles	148
Orbits – optic nerve	150

Parathyroid glands

PREPARATION
None.

POSITION
Supine.

PROBE
7.0–10.0 MHz linear transducer.

METHOD
Images are obtained in the longitudinal and transverse planes.

APPEARANCE
The four normal parathyroid glands are generally located at the poles of the thyroid lobes, although the inferior parathyroid glands may be ectopic, found in the upper mediastinum. Occasionally the normal parathyroid gland can be identified separate from thyroid tissue, especially in a longitudinal view. A linear high-reflective band representing an aponeurosis or a fibrous sheath may surround the gland. The normal parathyroid gland may either be seen as a slightly low-reflective or slightly high-reflective oval area adjacent to the normal thyroid. A parathyroid adenoma is identified as an oval shaped low-reflective area, with increased color Doppler flow, in the expected location of a parathyroid gland.

MEASUREMENTS
Average normal parathyroid measures 5 × 3 × 1 mm.

FURTHER READING
Reeder SB, Desser TS, Weigel RJ, Jeffrey RB. Sonography in primary hyperparathyroidism. Review with emphasis on scanning technique. *Journal of Ultrasound in Medicine* 2002;**21**:539–552.

Simeone JF, Mueller PR, Ferrucci JT Jr, van Sonnenberg E, Wang CA, Hall DA, Wittenberg J. High-resolution real-time sonography of the parathyroid. *Radiology* 1981;**141**:745–751.

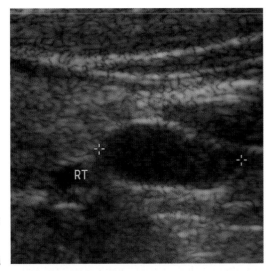

Figure 50a
Longitudinal plane demonstrating an oval low-reflective area (between cursors) surrounded by the high-reflective aponeurosis, characteristic of a parathyroid adenoma

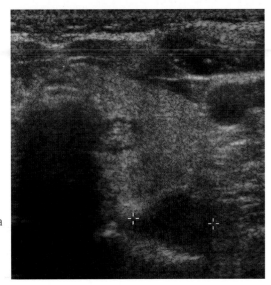

Figure 50b Same patient, with the parathyroid adenoma demonstrated in an axial plane, at the lower pole of the left lobe of the thyroid

Submandibular salivary glands

PREPARATION
None.

POSITION
Supine.

PROBE
7.5–10.0 MHz linear array probe.

METHOD
The gland is imaged in two planes: paramandibular and longitudinal planes.

APPEARANCE
Homogenous high-reflective parenchyma, well demarcated from the surrounding tissues.

MEASUREMENTS
Three measurements are obtained: anteroposterior and lateral–medial direction, and then depth. Volume is calculated as if gland is a spherical body, using the formula:

$$\text{volume (ml)} = (\pi \times \text{height} \times (\text{diameter})^2)/4$$

Normal values		
Anteroposterior length	Paramandibular length (depth)	Lateral–medial length
35 ± 5.7 mm	14.3 ± 2.9 mm	33.7 ± 5.4 mm

FURTHER READING
Dost P, Kaiser S. Ultrasonographic biometry in salivary glands.
Ultrasound in Medicine and Biology 1997;**23**:1299–1303.

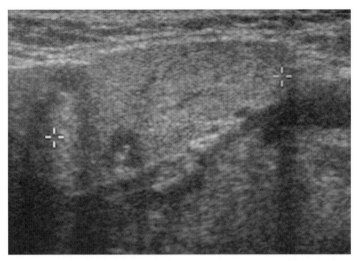

Figure 51a The submandibular gland viewed in a paramandibular section in order to measure the lateral-medial length

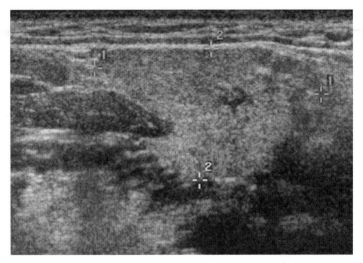

Figure 51b The submandibular gland viewed in a longitudinal plane in order to document the anteroposterior and depth measurements

Parotid salivary glands

PREPARATION
None.

POSITION
Supine.

PROBE
7.5–10.0 MHz linear array transducer.

METHOD
The gland is imaged in a transverse plane and in an axis parallel to the ramus of the mandible (parallel direction to the normal dental occlusion).

APPEARANCE
The gland is homogeneous and of high reflectivity, more so than that of the submandibular gland.

MEASUREMENTS

	Length (mean ± SD, mm)
Axis parallel to ramus of mandible	46.3 ± 7.7 mm
Dimension in transverse axis	37.4 ± 5.6 mm
Parotid parenchyma	
Lateral to mandible	7.4 ± 1.7 mm
Dorsal to mandible	22.8 ± 3.6 mm

FURTHER READING
Dost P, Kaiser S. Ultrasonographic biometry in salivary glands. *Ultrasound in Medicine and Biology* 1997;**23**:1299–1303.

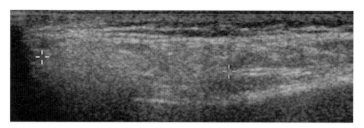

Figure 52a The parotid gland, homogeneous and high reflective, is imaged in a transverse plane

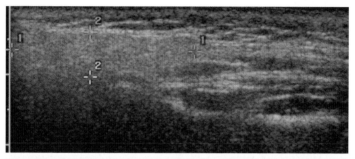

Figure 52b The parotid gland is also imaged in an axis parallel to the ramus of the mandible (parallel direction to the normal dental occlusion)

Thyroid gland

PREPARATION
None.

POSITION
Supine with the neck extended.

PROBE
7.5–10.0 MHz linear transducer.

METHOD
Longitudinal and transverse images obtained in the lower half of the neck from the midline.

APPEARANCE
Below the subcutaneous tissues is a 1–2 mm thin low-reflective line corresponding to the platysma muscle. Anterior to this is a thin high-reflective line representing the superficial cervical aponeurosis. The thyroid gland is made up of two lobes connected medially by the isthmus, which has a transverse course. A minority 10–40% of normal people have a third lobe (pyramidal) arising from the isthmus which runs upwards along the same longitudinal axis as the thyroid lobes but lies in front of the thyroid cartilage. Thyroid parenchyma has a fine homogeneous echo pattern, which is of higher reflectivity than the contiguous muscular structures and is interrupted at the periphery by the arterial and venous vessels.

MEASUREMENTS

Age	Length (mm)	Anteroposterior diameter (mm)
Newborn	18–20	8–9
1 year	25	12–15
Adult	40–60	13–20

- The mean thickness of the isthmus is 4–6 mm.
- Thyroid volume may be calculated using the right and left anteroposterior lobe measurements (RAP and LAP) by the following formula;

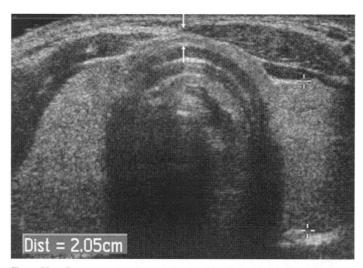

Figure 53a Transverse plane through the thyroid at the level of the thyroid isthmus, demonstrating a depth measurement of the left lobe. The arrows represent the depth of the isthmus

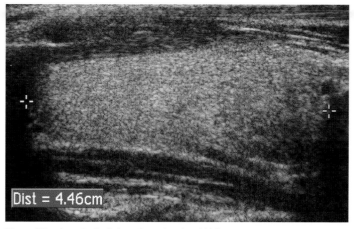

Figure 53b Longitudinal plane through a thyroid lobe

volume = $(6.91 \times RAP) + (3.05 \times LAP) - 3.48$

- The difference in thyroid volume between males and females is explained solely by a difference in body weight:
  male thyroid volume 19.6 ± 4.7 ml; female 17.5 ± 3.2 ml.

DOPPLER STUDIES OF THE THYROID ARTERIES

There are two thyroid arteries on each side, superior and inferior. Rarely a third artery is present in the midline, known as the arteria ima.

- Mean diameter of these vessels is 1–2 mm.
- Peak systolic velocity is 20–40 cm/s.
- End diastolic velocity is 10–15 cm/s.
  The thyroid veins originate from the perithyroid venous plexus and join to form three main groups, which drain into the ipsilateral jugular vein. The largest vessel is a lower vein and can measure up to 7–8 mm.

FURTHER READING

Hegedus L, Perrild H, Poulsen LR, Andersen JR, Holm B, Schnohr P, Jensen G, Hansen JM. The determination of thyroid volume by ultrasound and its relationship to body weight, age and sex in normal subjects. *Journal of Clinical Endocrinology and Metabolism* 1983;**56**:260–263.

Udea D. Normal volume of the thyroid gland in children. *Journal of Clinical Ultrasound* 1990;**18**:455–462.

Vade A, Gottschalk ME, Yetter EM, Subbaiah P. Sonographic measurements of the neonatal thyroid gland. *Journal of Ultrasound in Medicine* 1997;**16**:395–399.

Lymph nodes in the neck

PREPARATION
None.

POSITION
Supine.

PROBE
5.0–10.0 MHz linear transducer.

METHOD
Use the thyroid as a landmark and assess the anterior and posterior aspects of both sides of the neck.

APPEARANCE
Ultrasound features that should be assessed:

*   *Lymph node shape:* Assessed by measuring the longitudinal (L) and transverse (T) diameter on the same image and calculating the L/T ratio. This is normal when L/T >2, that is when the shape is oval. Another method is to measure the ratio of the minimal to maximum diameter of a node in the transverse plane. A ratio of more than 0.55 yields the highest accuracy when predicting malignancy with ultrasound.
*   *Nodal hilus:* This should be of high reflectivity and wide. The presence of hilar narrowing or cortical widening (either concentrically or eccentrically) should be regarded with suspicion for malignancy.
*   *Nodal size:* On ultrasound, this is not a reliable criterion for differentiating benign from malignant nodes.
*   *Calcification:* Calcification is found in a significantly lower number of malignant nodes.
*   Doppler waveforms: The resistance index can be measured, and a cut-off of 0.70 for differentiating benign (<0.70) from malignant but with considerable overlap in recordings.

Figure 54a
Longitudinal plane
through an oval lymph
node demonstrating
features of benign
disease. Longitudinal
(L) and transverse (T)
diameter on the same
image, calculating the
L/T ratio which is
normal when L/T >2

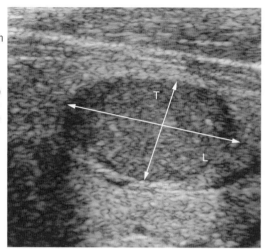

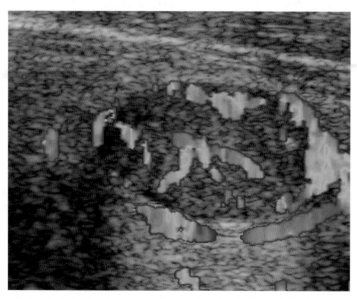

Figure 54b Color Doppler image of the same lymph node demonstrating hilar
vessel architecture

FURTHER READING

Na DG, Lim HK, Byun HS, Kim HD, Ko YH, Baek JH. Differential diagnosis of cervical lymphadenopathy: usefulness of color Doppler sonography. *American Journal of Roentgenology* 1997;**168**:1311–1316.

Takashima S, Sone S, Nomura N, Tomiyama N, Kobyashi T, Nakamura H. Nonpalpable lymph nodes of the neck: assessment with US and US-guided fine needle aspiration biopsy. *Journal of Clinical Ultrasound* 1997;**25**:283–292.

Vassallo P, Wernecke K, Roos N, Peters PE. Differentiation of benign from malignant superficial lymphadenopathy: the role of high resolution US. *Radiology* 1992;**183**:215–220.

Orbits – extraocular muscles

PREPARATION
None

POSITION
Supine in a reclining position with the eyelid closed.

PROBE
10 MHz linear transducer

METHOD
Transverse and longitudinal planes of the four recti are obtained. The recti muscles appear as low-reflective structures.

MEASUREMENTS

Muscle	Diameter in normal population (mm)	
	Mean ± SD	Median
Superior rectus	5.3 ± 0.7	5.4
Lateral rectus	3.0 ± 0.4	3.1
Inferior rectus	2.6 ± 0.5	2.6
Medial rectus	3.5 ± 0.6	3.6

FURTHER READING
Byrne SF, Gendron EK, Glaser JS, Feuer W, Atta H. Diameter of normal extraocular recti muscles with echography. *American Journal of Opthalmology* 1991;**112**:706–713.

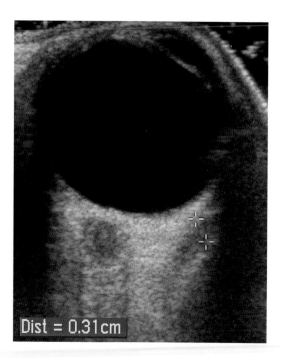

Figure 55 Axial plane image through the orbit, demonstrating the diameter of the medial rectus muscle

Orbits – optic nerve

PREPARATION
None.

POSITION
Supine in a reclining position, with eyelid closed.

PROBE
10 MHz linear transducer

APPEARANCE
Tubular structure. Homogenous, low-reflective, parallel nerve fibre bundle surrounded by a highly reflective dural sheath.

MEASUREMENTS
Optic nerve width 2.4 mm to 3.4 mm; median of 2.9 mm and no more than 0.3 mm between the two nerves.

FURTHER READING
Atta HR. Imaging of the optic nerve with standardized echography. *Eye* 1988;**2**:358–366.

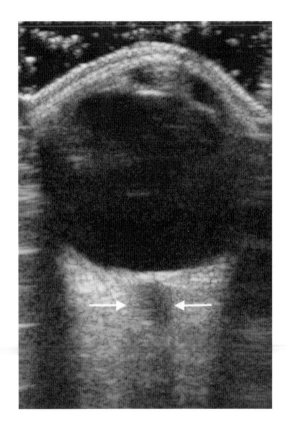

Figure 56 Axial plane image through the orbit, demonstrating the optic nerve (arrows)

7

NEONATAL BRAIN

Maria E.K. Sellars,
Wui K. Chong and
Paul S. Sidhu

Ventricular size   154
Doppler studies of intercranial
    blood flow   158

Ventricular size

PREPARATION
None.

POSITION
Supine.

PROBE
5.0–7.5 MHz curvilinear array transducer with a small footprint. A 10 MHz linear transducer will demonstrate the superficial subdural space.

METHOD
Performed through the anterior fontanell in the neonate where this remains patent. Posterior fontanelle allows access to the posterior brain structures. Oblique coronal and oblique sagittal views are obtained, and the frontal horns of the lateral ventricles are measured.

APPEARANCE
The ventricles are clearly identified as low reflective areas within the midlevel reflectivity of the brain parenchyma. The walls of the ventricles are well demonstrated in the premature infant, but are often opposed in the term infant. Measurements are taken in the coronal direction at the level of the foramen of Monro. A minor degree of asymmetry of the ventricles is common, the left being slightly larger. Serial measurements are important to document progression or regression.

MEASUREMENTS
Ventricular width:[1] Taken from the medial wall to the floor of the ventricle at the widest point, measured at 0 mm when the ventricle appears as a thin high-reflective line. This should be described as depth rather than width.

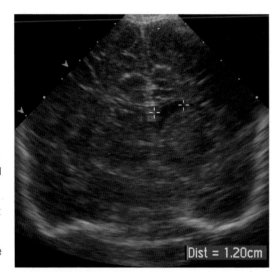

Dist = 1.20cm

Figure 57
Measurements are taken in the coronal direction at the level of the foramen of Monro. Ventricular width measurement is taken from the medial wall to the floor of the ventricle at the widest point

Gestational age (weeks)	Mean depth (mm)
26–27	0.9
28–29	1.01
30–31	1.32
32–33	1.05
34–35	0.82
36–37	0.74
38–39	1.02
40–41	0.91
42	1.09

Ventricular ratio (VR):[2] Using a transverse approach, from the temporal window (or lateral fontalle), the ventricular width (VW), from the midline to the lateral ventricle wall and the hemispheric width (HW) from the midline to the inner skull margin are used to calculate the VR (VR = VW/HW).

	Term neonates Mean (range) (cm)	Premature neonates Mean (range) (cm)
Lateral ventricle width (VW)	1.1 (0.9–1.3)	1.0 (0.5–1.3)
Hemisphere width (HW)	3.9 (3.1–4.7)	3.1 (2.1–4.3)
Ventricular–hemisphere ratio (VW/HW)	28% (24–30%)	31% (24–34%)

- The upper limit of normal for ventricular depth measured in the coronal plane is 1.3 cm for a single ventricle or 2.5 cm for both measured together.

REFERENCES

1. Perry RN, Bowman ED, Murton LJ, Roy RN, de Crespigny LC. Ventricular size in newborn infants. *Journal of Ultrasound in Medicine* 1985;**4**:475–477.
2. Johnson ML, Mack LA, Rumack CM, Frost M, Rashbaum C. B-mode echoencephalography in the normal and high-risk infant. *American Journal of Roentgenology* 1979;**133**:375–381.

FURTHER READING

Poland RL, Slovis TL, Shankaran S. Normal values for ventricular size as determined by real time sonographic techniques. *Pediatric Radiology* 1985;**15**:12–14.

Doppler studies of intercranial blood flow

PREPARATION
None.

POSITION
- *Through the anterior fontanelle:* Sagittal and angled/sagittal or coronal and angled/coronal views.
- *Through the temporal bone:* Axial image with transducer placed 1 cm anterior and superior to tragus of the ear.

PROBE
Linear 7.5 MHz transducer.

METHOD
Resistance indices (RI) are obtained from middle cerebral (MCA), anterior cerebral (ACA), internal carotid (ICA) and posterior cerebral arteries.

APPEARANCE
The ACAs and ICAs course parallel to the image plane on trans-fontanellar views, providing the optimum Doppler angle. For the same reason, the MCAs are best visualized on the transtemporal view.

MEASUREMENTS

	RI
Anterior cerebral artery (premature)	0.5–1.0
Anterior, middle and posterior cerebral arteries (term)	0.6–0.8
Internal carotid artery (term)	0.5–0.8

- Intracranial RI normally decrease with increasing gestational age.[1]
- Elevated or rising RI is seen in hydrocephalus and cerebral edema due to hypoxic-ischemic brain injury.
- Low RI is seen in babies on extracorporeal membrane oxygenation (ECMO).

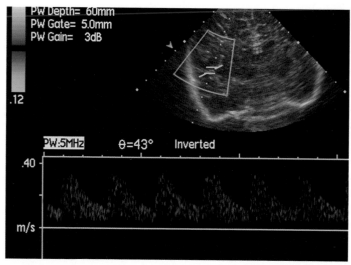

Figure 58 A coronal image through the anterior fontanelle with a spectral Doppler waveform obtained from the middle cerebral artery from which the resistance index may be calculated

REFERENCE

1. Horgan JG, Rumack CM, Hay T, Manco-Johnson ML, Merenstein GB, Esola C. Absolute intracranial blood-flow velocities evaluated by duplex Doppler sonography in asymptomatic preterm and term neonates. *American Journal of Roentgenology* 1989;**152**:1059–1064.

FURTHER READING

Raju TN, Zikos E. Regional cerebral blood velocity in infants. A real-time transcranial and fontanellar pulsed Doppler study. *Journal of Ultrasound in Medicine* 1987;**6**:497–507.

8 GASTROINTESTINAL TRACT

Zelena A. Aziz,
Keshthra Satchithananda,
Maria E.K. Sellars and
Paul S. Sidhu

Pyloric stenosis	162
Appendix	164
Upper gastrointestinal tract wall – endoscopic ultrasound	166
Bowel wall – transabdominal ultrasound	168
Anal endosonography	170

Pyloric stenosis

PREPARATION
No feed for at least 2 hours.

POSITION
Supine, left anterior oblique, or right decubitus.

PROBE
5.0–7.5 MHz curvilinear transducer or a 5.0–7.0 MHz linear transducer.

METHOD
Longitudinal and transverse preliminary views right of midline at level of subxiphoid space. The infant is usually bottle fed at the time of the examination. Image with patient right side down and obtain longitudinal and transverse views as before.

APPEARANCE
Thickened muscle is seen as a low-reflective layer, superficial to the high-reflective mucosal layer. In transverse plane, the canal resembles a doughnut, medial to the gallbladder and anterior to the right kidney. There is an absence of peristalsis.

MEASUREMENTS

Pylorus	mm
Diameter	≥15
Length	≥17
Muscle thickness	≥4

FURTHER READING
Haller JO, Cohen HL. Hypertrophic pyloric stenosis: diagnosis using US. *Radiology* 1986;**161**:335–339.
O'Keeffe FN, Stansberry SD, Swischuk LE, Hayden CK Jr. Antropyloric muscle thickness at US in infants: what is normal? *Radiology* 1991;**178**:827–830.

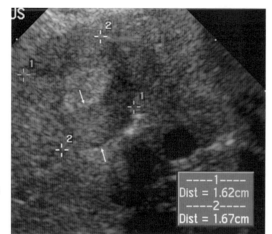

Figure 59a Axial plane through the pylorus demonstrating the 'doughnut' appearance, with the arrows indicating the low-reflective muscle layer

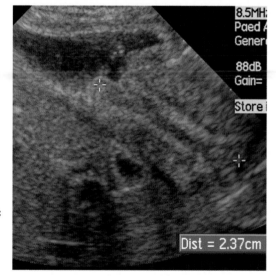

Figure 59b Pyloric length measured in the longitudinal plane (right decubitus position)

Appendix

PREPARATION
Full bladder. After a 10-minute search for the appendix on full bladder and if this is negative, ask the patient to empty the bladder and continue the search.

POSITION
Supine and left lateral decubitus position if retrocaval appendix is suspected.

PROBE
5.0 MHz linear array transducer or a 5.0–7.0 MHz curvilinear transducer.

METHOD
Place transducer transversely below edge of right hepatic lobe, in front of the right kidney and move slowly down to right iliac fossa along line of the ascending colon. Identifying the caecum and then trace the appendix, which is draped over the right iliac vessels anterior to the ileopsoas muscle.

APPEARANCE
Features of normal appendix are:
- A compressible blind-ended tubular structure.
- Surrounded by normal appearing fat.
- Wall thickness <3 mm, measured from the serosa to the lumen and diameter measurement of <6 mm, measured from serosa to serosa.

MEASUREMENTS
Appendicitis is characterized by a wall thickness >3 mm and a diameter >6 mm. Hypervascular wall with color Doppler, free fluid and presence of an appendicolith, are secondary signs of appendicitis.

FURTHER READING
Quillin SQ, Siegel MJ. Appendicitis: Efficacy of color Doppler sonography. *Radiology* 1994;**191**:557–560.
Rioux M. Sonographic detection of normal and abnormal appendix. *American Journal of Roentgenology* 1992;**158**:773–778.

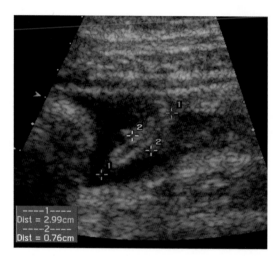

Figure 60 A tubular structure representing the appendix is surrounded by low-reflective fluid

Upper gastrointestinal tract wall – endoscopic ultrasound

This is a specialized procedure and is carried out in a similar manner to standard upper gastrointestinal endoscopy.

PREPARATION
The patient is sedated and given pharyngeal local anaesthesia.

POSITION
Left lateral position.

PROBE
An ultrasonic endoscope consisting of a 7.5 MHz ultrasound mechanical sector-scan transducer housed in an oil-filled chamber at the tip of a specially adapted fibreoptic endoscope.

METHOD
After introduction of the endoscope to the desired position under direct vision, intraluminal gas is aspirated.

Three methods are available for exploration of the upper GI tract wall:
- Direct apposition of the transducer on the mucosa: used for oesophagus.
- Contact of a small balloon filled with water over the tip of the ultrasonic probe: used for oesophagus, gastric and duodenal walls.
- Direct instillation of deaerated water, usually about 500 ml: for gastric and duodenal walls.

APPEARANCE
The ultrasound beam passing through the gastrointestinal wall will potentially encounter six interfaces between tissue layers, which allows the visualization of five separate layers. These layers have their respective histological correlates.

Layer 1	High-reflective line	Luminal/mucosa
Layer 2	Low reflectivity	Deep mucosa
Layer 3	High reflectivity	Submucosa
Layer 4	Low reflectivity	Muscularis propria
Layer 5	High reflectivity	Adventitia/serosa

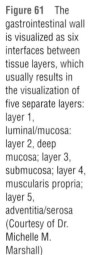

Figure 61 The gastrointestinal wall is visualized as six interfaces between tissue layers, which usually results in the visualization of five separate layers: layer 1, luminal/mucosa: layer 2, deep mucosa; layer 3, submucosa; layer 4, muscularis propria; layer 5, adventitia/serosa (Courtesy of Dr. Michelle M. Marshall)

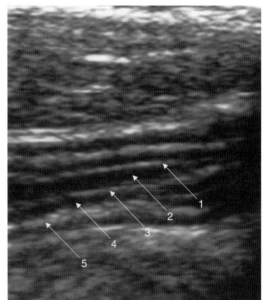

FURTHER READING

Caletti GC, Bolondi L, Zani L, Labo G. Technique of endoscopic ultrasonography investigation: Esophagus, stomach and duodenum. *Scandinavian Journal of Gastroenterology* 1986;**21**:1–5.

Kimmey MB, Martin RW, Haggitt RC, Wang KY, Franklin DW, Silverstein FE. Histologic correlates of gastrointestinal ultrasound images. *Gastroenterology* 1989;**96**:433–441.

Shorvon PJ, Lees WR, Frost RA, Cotton PB. Upper gastrointestinal endoscopic ultrasonography in gastroenterology. *British Journal of Radiology* 1987;**60**:429–438.

Bowel wall – transabdominal ultrasound

PREPARATION
None.

POSITION
Supine.

PROBE
3.5–5.0 MHz curvilinear transducer.

METHOD
Bowel wall thickness may be measured before and after ingestion of water. Measurements should be made only on images obtained in transverse sections. In the non-distended state bowel segments demonstrate a target configuration. The thickness of bowel wall is measured from the edge of the high-reflective core representing the intraluminal gas and mucus, to the outer border of the low-reflective representing the bowel wall. In the distended state (following ingestion of water), the lumen is fluid filled. Distension is considered adequate when the luminal diameter is greater than 8 cm for the stomach, 3 cm for the small bowel and 5 cm for the large bowel. Measurements should be made from the low-reflective intraluminal fluid to the interface representing the serosa.

APPEARANCE
Although it has been shown that the thickness of the bowel wall depends on the amount of distension of the bowel segment, pathologic thickening of the bowel wall should be suspected when it measures more than 5 mm.

MEASUREMENT

| | Average wall thickness (range, mm) | |
	Non-distended	Distended
Stomach	5 (2–6)	4 (2–4)
Small bowel	3 (2–3)	3 (2–3)
Large bowel	6 (4–9)	3 (2–4)

FURTHER READING
Fleischer AC, Muhletaler CA, James AE Jr. Sonographic assessment of the bowel wall. *American Journal of Roentgenology* 1981;**136**:887–891.

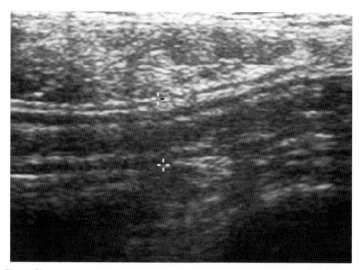

Figure 62a
Normal transverse
colon (between
cursors) with no
fecal residue present

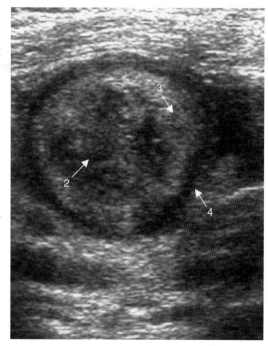

Figure 62b
Transverse plane not
at an absolute right
angle (layers 1 and 5
not visualized) but
demonstrating layer
2, deep mucosa;
layer 3, submucosa;
and layer 4,
muscularis propria
(Courtesy of Dr.
Michelle M.
Marshall)

Anal endosonography

PREPARATION
None.

POSITION
Left lateral position. Females should be examined prone due to the symmetry of the anterior perineal structures in this position.

PROBE
A high frequency (7–10 MHz) rotating rectal probe is used which provides a 360° image. A hard sonolucent plastic cone covers the transducer and is filled with degassed water for acoustic coupling. The cone is covered with a condom with ultrasound gel applied to both surfaces.

METHOD
Serial images are obtained on slow withdrawal of the probe down the anal canal, images are typically taken at the upper, mid and lower anal canal.

APPEARANCE
The normal anal canal is composed of five distinct layers: the mucosa, the submucosa, internal anal sphincter, the intersphincteric plane and external anal sphincter.

- *Mucosa:* This low-reflective layer is immediately adjacent to the probe and is continuous with the rectal mucosa.
- *Submucosa:* This high-reflective layer lies between the mucosa and the internal anal sphincter, becoming progressively thicker and denser caudally.
- *Internal anal sphincter:* The smooth muscle of the internal sphincter is seen as a homogeneous low-reflective circular band >2–3 mm in width, extending caudally to a level just proximal to the anal verge. The thickness should be measured at the 3 o'clock or 9 o'clock positions.
- *Intersphincteric:* This is a narrow high-reflective band between the two sphincter planes.
- *External anal sphincter (EAS):* The striated muscle of the external anal sphincter has mixed reflectivity and a linear pattern, giving a streaky appearance. The EAS can be traced from the puborectalis component of the levator ani muscle to its cutaneous termination. The EAS is consistent in appearance for both sexes posterolaterally. However, anteriorly, in females, the muscle is deficient in the

immediate region of the perineal body and vagina. In males, the sphincter tapers anteriorly into two arcs that meet in the midline.

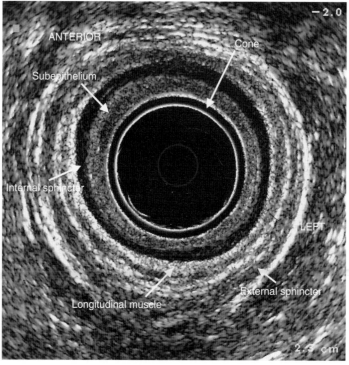

Figure 63 The normal anal canal is composed of five distinct layers: mucosa, submucosa, internal anal sphincter, the intersphincteric plane, and external anal sphincter (Courtesy of Dr. Michelle M. Marshall)

FURTHER READING

Law PJ, Bartram CI. Anal endosonography: technique and normal anatomy. *Gastrointestinal Radiology* 1989;**14**:349–353.

9

MUSCULOSKELETAL SYSTEM

*Keshthra Satchithananda and
David Elias*

General considerations	174
Upper limb – shoulder	176
Long head of biceps	176
Subscapularis tendon	178
Supraspinatus tendon	180
Infraspinatus tendon	182
Upper limb – elbow	184
Anterior joint space	184
Olecranon fossa	186
Lateral elbow	188
Medial elbow	190
Upper limb – wrist	192
Dorsal tendons	192
Carpal tunnel	194
Lower limb – hips	196
Hip effusion	196
Developmental dysplasia of the hip	198
Lower limb – knee	200
Lower limb – ankle	202
Anterior, medial, lateral tendons	202
Achilles tendon	204
Lower limb – foot	206
Plantar fascia	206
Interdigital web spaces	208

GENERAL CONSIDERATIONS

PREPARATION
None.

POSITION
See individual examinations.

PROBE
- High resolution, high quality ultrasound equipment.
- >10 MHz linear transducer for small superficial structures.
- 7–15 MHz linear transducers for tendons of extremities.
- 3.5–7 MHz linear/curvilinear transducers to image large or deep muscles.

Linear probes ideal to provide uniform field of view with superior near-field resolution.

METHOD
See individual examinations.

APPEARANCE
- *Muscle bundles:* Are low-reflective with high-reflective intramuscular fibroadipose septa, perimuscular epimysium and intermuscular fascia.
- *Tendons:* Consist of parallel fascicles of collagen fibres, which appear as parallel high-reflective lines due to multiple reflective interfaces. Most tendons are lined by a synovial sheath, which contains a thin film of fluid. This appears as a low-reflective rim normally <2 mm thick. Those without a sheath (e.g. tendo Achilles) have a surrounding high-reflective line due to the dense connective tissue of the epitendineum.
- *Ligaments:* Have more interwoven and irregular collagen fibres than tendons and thus appear as 2–3 mm thick homogeneous high-reflective bands.
- *Bursa:* A normal bursa appears as a low-reflective line representing fluid surrounded by a high-reflective line.
- *Peripheral nerves:* Exhibit parallel linear internal echoes on longitudinal images. On transverse images nerves are round or oval structures with tiny punctate internal echoes. Nerves do not move with flexion or extension of the regional muscles.

MEASUREMENTS
See individual examinations

ARTIFACTS
Anisotropic structures demonstrate different characteristics depending upon the direction from which they are evaluated. Tendons are markedly anisotropic; nerves, muscles and ligaments less so. Thus, for tendons in particular, the angle of insonation must remain perpendicular to the imaged structure to demonstrate its normal high-reflective ultrasound appearance. Loss of perpendicularity results in artifactual low reflectivity. For superficial tendons with a curved overlying skin surface, the use of a standoff pad, or imaging of structures in a water bath (e.g. for finger tendons) can be helpful to allow maintenance of probe contact with the skin and at the same time keep a perpendicular insonation angle. Alternatively, modern units, which allow beam steering or compound imaging, may be helpful in reducing the anisotropy artefact.

UPPER LIMB – SHOULDER

Long head of biceps

POSITION
Patient is imaged while sitting on a revolving chair or stool. Humerus internally rotated 10–20° with elbow flexed and hand, with palm up, resting on patient's lap.

PROBE
7.0–10.0 MHz linear transducer.

METHOD
Transducer placed transversely and longitudinally across bicipital groove.

APPEARANCE
- *Transverse section:* The biceps tendon is a high-reflective oval structure within bicipital groove. Important view to detect intra-articular fluid.
- *Longitudinal section:* Should identify fibrillary echo pattern of tendon. Measurements are made in the transverse plane of the width of long head of biceps within the bicipital groove.

MEASUREMENTS

	Right (mean ± SD)	Left (mean ± SD)
Male	3.2 ± 0.5 mm	3.3 ± 0.4 mm
Female	2.7 ± 0.3 mm	3.0 ± 0.3 mm

FURTHER READING
Middleton WD, Teefey SA, Yamaguchi K. Sonography of the shoulder. *Seminars in Musculoskeletal Radiology* 1998;**211**:211–222.

Van Holsbeeck MV, Introcaso JH. Appendix: table of normal values. In: van Holsbeeck MV, Introcaso JH. eds. *Muscloskeletal Ultrasound*, 2nd edn. Mosby-Year Book, St. Louis, 2001, pp. 625–628.

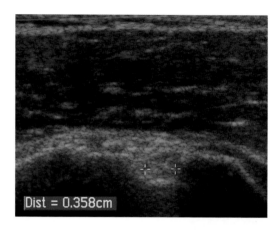

Figure 64
Transverse image
through the biceps
tendon in the
bicipital groove
(cursors)

Subscapularis tendon

POSITION

Patient is imaged while sitting on a revolving chair or stool. Humerus externally rotated to stretch the subscapularis tendon.

PROBE

7.0–10.0 MHz linear transducer.

METHOD

Transducer placed transversely and longitudinally across the subscapularis tendon, which lies medial to the bicipital groove inserting into the lesser tuberosity.

APPEARANCE

Subscapularis tendon has a convex margin superficially and follows the convex humeral cortex on its deep aspect. Transversely the multipenate anatomy of the tendon may be appreciated. Small subdeltoid effusions may be apparent superficial to subscapularis.

FURTHER READING

Middleton WD, Teefey SA, Yamaguchi K. Sonography of the shoulder. *Seminars in Musculoskeletal Radiology* 1998;**211**:211–222.

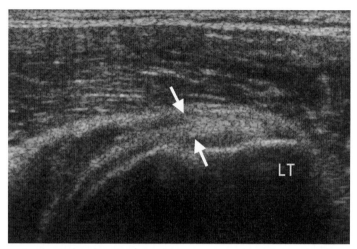

Figure 65 Subscapularis tendon has a convex margin superficially and follows the convex humeral cortex on its deep aspect (between arrows)

Supraspinatus tendon

POSITION
Patient is imaged while sitting on a revolving chair or stool. Humerus extended and internally rotated; 'hand in opposite back pocket'.

PROBE
7.0–10.0 MHz linear transducer.

METHOD
Transducer placed transversely and longitudinally across shoulder joint.

APPEARANCE
- *Transverse section:* High-reflectivity fibrillary pattern of tendon fibres with a smoothly convex superficial contour deep to deltoid and subdeltoid fat stripe. The tendon lies superficial to the low-reflective cartilage of the humeral head.
- *Longitudinal section:* Tendon is thick as it emerges from under the acromion and thins distally as it inserts into the greater tuberosity. This results in a triangular shape.

FURTHER READING
Middleton WD, Teefey SA, Yamaguchi K. Sonography of the shoulder. *Seminars in Musculoskeletal Radiology* 1998;**211**:211–222.

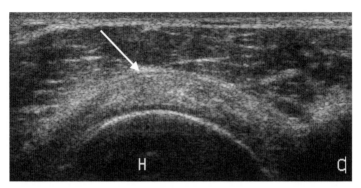

Figure 66a Transverse view of the supraspinatus tendon (arrow) as it passes over the humerus (H). Note the coracoid process (C)

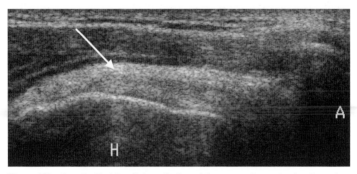

Figure 66b Longitudinal (mediolateral) view of the supraspinatus tendon (arrow), as it passes beneath the acromion (A) and over the humerus (H)

Infraspinatus tendon

POSITION
Patient is imaged while sitting on a revolving chair or stool. Ipsilateral hand is placed on the contralateral shoulder to stretch out infraspinatus. Probe placed on the posterior shoulder, inferior and parallel to the scapular spine, sweeping laterally to identify the muscle belly and then tendon.

PROBE
7.0–10.0 MHz linear transducer.

METHOD
Transducer placed transversely and longitudinally across infraspinatus.

APPEARANCE
Infraspinatus tendon appears as elongated soft tissue triangle that attaches to greater tuberosity of the humerus. The infraspinatus tendon needs to be differentiated from teres minor tendon. The latter is inferior to the infraspinatus tendon and appears trapezoidal with internal echoes that run in oblique lines as opposed to horizontal lines of infraspinatus tendon.

FURTHER READING
Middleton WD, Teefey SA, Yamaguchi K. Sonography of the shoulder. *Seminars in Musculoskeletal Radiology* 1998;**211**:211–222.

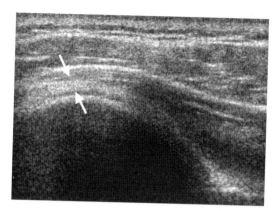

Figure 67
Longitudinal view through the infraspinatus tendon (arrows)

UPPER LIMB – ELBOW

Anterior joint space

POSITION
Patient lying or seated with forearm supinated and elbow extended.

PROBE
7.0–10.0 MHz linear transducer.

METHOD
Transducer placed longitudinally along anterior radio-capitellar joint.
Identify anterior synovial recess.

APPEARANCE
The anterior capsule of elbow joint is a high-reflective line that follows
the ventral contours of the proximal radial head and distal humeral
capitellum. Between the capsule and the bone lies a 1 mm thick low-
reflective layer representing articular cartilage which should not be
mistaken for abnormal joint fluid.

FURTHER READING
Hashimoto BE, Kramer DJ, Wiitala L. Applications of
  musculoskeletal sonography. *Journal of Clinical Ultrasound*
  1999;**27**:293–318.

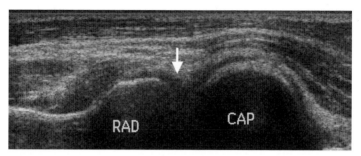

Figure 68 Transverse view through the anterior joint space of the elbow (RAD, radius; CAP, capitellum). The arrow points to the anterior synovial recess, where the joint may be evaluated for the presence of an effusion

Olecranon fossa

POSITION
Patient's elbow is flexed at 90°.

PROBE
7.0–10.0 MHz linear transducer.

METHOD
Transducer placed longitudinally and transversely across the olecranon fossa.

APPEARANCE
Within the olecranon fossa is the posterior fat pad. The fibrous joint capsule is a high-reflective line superficial to the fat pad and the trochlea.

FURTHER READING
Hashimoto BE, Kramer DJ, Wiitala L. Applications of
   musculoskeletal sonography. *Journal of Clinical Ultrasound*
   1999;**27**:293–318.

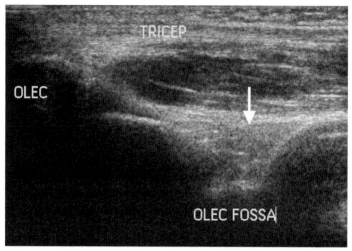

Figure 69 Longitudinal view through the olecranon fossa. The arrow points to the posterior fat pad (OLEC, olecranon; OLEC FOSSA, olecranon fossa; TRICEP, triceps tendon)

Lateral elbow

POSITION
Patient's elbows are extended with the palms of both hands together.

PROBE
7.0–10.0 MHz linear transducer.

METHOD
Transducer placed in longitudinal oblique direction on the lateral side of elbow.

APPEARANCE
The common forearm extensor tendon arises from the lateral epicondyle of the humerus. The radial collateral ligament lies deep to the tendon and attaches to the annular ligament at the radial head. The lateral ulnar collateral ligament forms a sling around the posterior radial neck to insert into the proximal ulna. These ligaments may be followed from their origin at the lateral epicondyle.

FURTHER READING
Hashimoto BE, Kramer DJ, Wiitala L. Applications of musculoskeletal sonography. *Journal of Clinical Ultrasound* 1999;**27**:293–318.

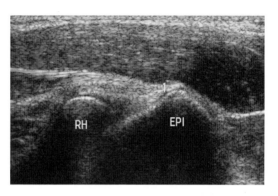

Figure 70 The common forearm extensor tendon (1) arises from the lateral epicondyle of the humerus (EPI) and lies superior to the radial head (RH)

Medial elbow

POSITION
Forearm placed in supination.

PROBE
7.0–10.0 MHz linear transducer.

METHOD
Transducer placed in longitudinal oblique position at the medial elbow joint.

APPEARANCE
The common flexor tendon arises at the medial epicondyle of the humerus. The anterior band of the ulnar collateral ligament arises from the medial epicondyle of the humerus and inserts on the medial coronoid process of the ulna. The posterior and oblique bands are less functionally important.

FURTHER READING
Hashimoto BE, Kramer DJ, Wiitala L. Applications of musculoskeletal sonography. *Journal of Clinical Ultrasound* 1999;**27**:293–318.

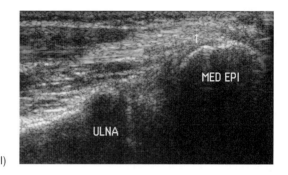

Figure 71 The common flexor tendon (1) arises from the medial epicondyle of the humerus (MED EPI)

UPPER LIMB – WRIST

Dorsal tendons

POSITION
Palm face down on examination table.

PROBE
7.0–10.0 MHz linear transducer.

METHOD
Transducer placed transversely across wrist at the level of the dorsal radial tubercle, and then moved to follow individual tendons in longitudinal and transverse section.

APPEARANCE
The dorsal tendons course through six separate synovial compartments. The dorsal radial tubercle acts as an anatomical landmark separating extensor pollicis longus, which lies on its ulnar side, from extensor carpi radialis brevis and longus, which lie on its radial side.

Radial side	Abductor pollicis longus tendon (volar aspect of anatomical snuffbox) and extensor pollicus brevis tendon (base of anatomical snuffbox)
↓	Extensor carpi radialis longus and extensor carpi radialis brevis tendons
Ulnar side	Extensor pollicus longus tendon (dorsal aspect of anatomical snuffbox)
	Extensor digitorum and extensor indicis tendons
	Extensor digiti minimi tendon
	Extensor carpi ulnaris tendon lying in a groove on the medial ulna

FURTHER READING
Hashimoto BE, Kramer DJ, Wiitala L. Applications of musculoskeletal sonography. *Journal of Clinical Ultrasound* 1999;27:293–318.

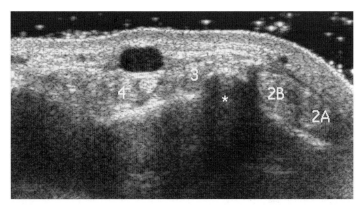

(a)

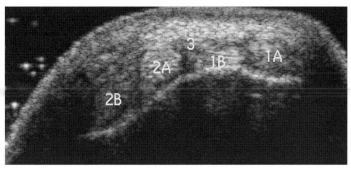

(b)

Figure 72 Transverse images through the dorsal wrist (a) at the level of the dorsal radial tubercle (*), and (b) approximately 1 cm beyond the dorsal radial tubercle and to its radial side. A prominent subcutaneous vein is noted superficial to extensor digitorum tendons. 1A, abductor pollicis longus tendon; 1B, extensor pollicus brevis tendon; 2A, extensor carpi radialis longus tendon; 2B, extensor carpi radialis brevis tendon; 3, extensor pollicus longus tendon; 4, extensor digitorum and extensor indicis tendons

Carpal tunnel

POSITION
Ventral side to evaluate carpal tunnel.

PROBE
7.0–10.0 MHz linear transducer

APPEARANCE
The floor of the carpal tunnel is formed by the carpal bones and its roof by the flexor retinaculum which attaches to the scaphoid tubercle and the trapezium laterally and the pisiform and hook of hamate medially. The median nerve lies just deep to the retinaculum at the radial aspect of the carpal tunnel. Also within the tunnel lie the flexor digitorum superficialis and profundus tendons and within its radial aspect, flexor pollicis longus and flexor carpi radialis. Superficial to the ulnar side of the carpal tunnel lies Guyon's canal containing the ulna nerve and artery. Flexor carpi ulnaris lies medially and inserts into the pisiform.

Identification of the median nerve is aided by noting that in the distal forearm it lies deep to flexor digitorum superficialis, and more distally it courses around the radial aspect of these tendons to reach the superficial carpal tunnel. Additionally it shows less movement on finger flexion/extension than the flexor tendons.

In carpal tunnel syndrome, wasting of the nerve as it passes into the carpal tunnel, palmar bowing of the flexor retinaculum and swelling of the nerve proximally may be identified. The cross-sectional area of the nerve should be measured at the distal carpal crease (i.e. the level of the pisiform and scaphoid tubercle). The wrist should be in a neutral position for a reproducible measurement.

MEASUREMENT

Normal cross-sectional area (mean $\pm$ SD, mm^2)	
Male	**Female**
8.3 ($\pm$1.9)	9.3 ($\pm$2.3)

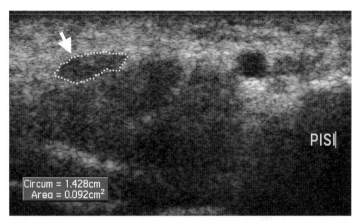

Figure 73 Transverse image obtained at the distal radial crease to demonstrate the pisiform (PISI), and circumferential area measurement of the median nerve (arrow)

FURTHER READING

Buchberger W, Judmaier W, Birbamer G, Lener M, Schmidauer C. Carpal tunnel syndrome: diagnosis with high-resolution sonography. *American Journal of Roentgenology* 1992;**159**:793–798.

Hashimoto BE, Kramer DJ, Wiitala L. Applications of musculoskeletal sonography. *Journal of Clinical Ultrasound* 1999;**27**:293–318.

Lee DH, van Holsbeeck MT, Janevski PK, Ganos DL, Ditmars DM, Darian VB. Diagnosis of carpal tunnel syndrome: ultrasound versus electromyography. *Radiographic Clinics of North America* 1999;**37**:859–872.

LOWER LIMB – HIPS

Hip effusion

POSITION
Supine with hip extended and slightly abducted.

PROBE
3.0–7.0 MHz linear or curvilinear transducer (dependent on patient age).

METHOD
Transducer placed along the length of the femoral neck.

APPEARANCE
The high-reflective anterior capsule is identified anterior to the femoral neck. Separation of the capsule from the femoral neck is normally 2–4 mm, and a difference of 2 mm or more between symptomatic and asymptomatic sides is considered significant for a joint effusion.

FURTHER READING
Nimityongskul P, McBryde AM, Jr., Anderson LD, Crotty JM.
  Ultrasonography in the management of painful hips in children.
  American Journal of Orthopedics 1996;**25**:411–414.

Figure 74
Longitudinal section through the anterior recess over the femoral head (FH) demonstrating normal appearances with no evidence of a hip effusion. The arrow indicates the position most likely for fluid to accumulate

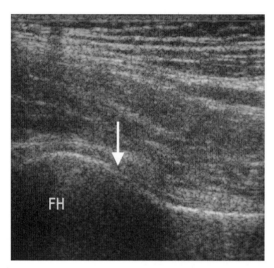

Developmental dysplasia of the hip

POSITION
Right and left lateral decubitus position for examination of each hip.

PROBE
Linear transducer; 7.5 MHz (newborn), 5–7.5 MHz (3 months).

METHOD
Infant should be as relaxed as possible (recent feed, parental presence and examination in a darkened room are helpful). Each position is assessed in the coronal and axial planes by placing the transducer longitudinally and transversely at the lateral hip. A static examination may be performed with the hip in the extended and 90° flexed positions. For dynamic examination the hip is flexed at 90° and gently adducted and abducted, and gentle posteriorly directed stress is applied to the flexed, adducted hip.

APPEARANCE
On coronal images the iliac wing is seen as a horizontal high-reflective line paralleling the transducer. The bony acetabulum forms a high-reflective curve medially with a defect representing the normal triradiate cartilage. Before ossification the femoral head is low-reflective with scattered specular echoes due to vascular channels. Superolateral to the femoral head the joint capsule is seen as a high-reflective line attaching to the ilium. Just deep to this a small high-reflective focus represents condensed fibrocartilage at the labral tip. The remaining labrum is low-reflective cartilage similar in reflectivity to the femoral head. On transverse images in hip flexion, the low-reflective femoral head lies within a 'V' shape formed by the femoral metaphysis anteriorly and the ischial part of the acetabulum posteriorly.

MEASUREMENTS
- *Graf alpha angle:* The angle between the iliac line and a line along the osseous acetabular roof on a coronal image of the hip. Normal is >60°.
- Percentage of the femoral head diameter covered by the bony acetabulum. Normal is >58%.

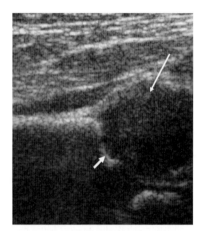

Figure 75a
Coronal section through the hip demonstrating the femoral head (long arrow) within the normal acetabulum (short arrow)

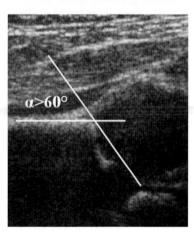

Figure 75b
Coronal section through the hip demonstrating the measurement of the alpha angle

FURTHER READING

Graf R. Fundamentals of sonographic diagnosis of infant hip dysplasia. *Journal of Pediatric Orthopedics* 1984;**4**:735–740.

Morin C, Harcke HT, MacEwen GD. The infant hip: real-time US assessment of acetabular development. *Radiology* 1985; **157**:673–677.

LOWER LIMB – KNEE

POSITION
Supine for anterior structures; knee extended for assessment of collateral ligaments. Quadriceps and patellar tendons are examined in flexion and extension. Measurement of fluid in the suprapatellar pouch should be performed with the knee flexed at 30°. Prone with the knee extended for assessment of the popliteal fossa.

PROBE
5.0–10.0 MHz linear transducer.

METHOD
The presence of joint fluid should be sought in the suprapatellar bursa and the medial and lateral joint recesses. The quadriceps and patellar tendons, medial and lateral collateral ligaments, the popliteal vessels and any cysts about the knee are evaluated in axial and longitudinal planes. Doppler and colour flow are used to assess the popliteal vessels.

APPEARANCE
- The suprapatellar pouch is a low-reflective band above the patella and deep to the quadriceps tendon. It lies between the suprapatellar and pre-femoral fat pads. At 30° of knee flexion it should be less than 4 mm thick.
- The medial collateral ligament has superficial and deep components. The superficial ligament attaches to the medial epicondyle of the femur and the medial tibial metaphysis and should measure no more than 5 mm thick proximally and no more than 3 mm thick distally.
- The lateral ligamentous structures include the iliotibial band anteriorly, which inserts onto the anterolateral tibia, the fibular collateral ligament which runs obliqely from the lateral epicondyle of the femur to insert on to the fibular head in conjuction with the distal tendon of biceps femoris, and the popliteus tendon which attaches to the popliteal notch of the lateral femur.

MEASUREMENTS

	Length (mean ± SD, mm)	
	Males	Females
Distal quadriceps tendon	5.1 ± 0.6	4.9 ± 0.6
Mid patellar tendon	3.1 ± 0.4	2.9 ± 0.5

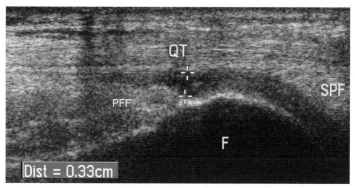

Figure 76a   Longitudinal view through the quadriceps tendon (QT), which lies anterior to the distal femur (F). The thickness of the suprapatellar pouch is measured (between cursors). Note that this joint recess lies between the suprapatellar fat (SPF) and the prefemoral fat (PFF)

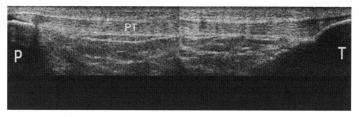

Figure 76b   Longitudinal view of the patellar tendon (PT) extending from the patella (P) to its insertion at the tibial tuberosity (T)

FURTHER READING

Hashimoto BE, Kramer DJ, Wiitala L. Applications of musculoskeletal sonography. *Journal of Clinical Ultrasound* 1999;**27**:293–318.

Van Holsbeeck MV, Introcaso JH. Appendix: table of normal values. In: van Holsbeeck MV, Introcaso JH. eds. *Muscloskeletal Ultrasound*, 2nd edn. Mosby-Year Book, St. Louis, 2001, pp. 625–628.

LOWER LIMB – ANKLE

Anterior, medial, lateral tendons

POSITION
Supine.

PROBE
7.0–10.0 MHz linear transducer.

METHOD
With the patient supine, the transducer is placed longitudinally across the tibiotalar joint to assess for fluid in the anterior recess. With the transducer placed transversely behind the lateral malleolus the peroneal tendons are identified (peroneus brevis lies anteromedially to longus). On a transverse image at the medial ankle tibialis posterior is identified just behind the malleolus and flexor digitorum longus lies just posterior to this. Flexor hallucis longus lies deep and may be more readily identified by a posterior approach. Anterior to the tibiotalar joint the three tendons identified (medial to lateral) are tibialis anterior, extensor hallucis longus and extensor digitorum longus. Each tendon is then followed in transverse and longitudinal section through its length.

APPEARANCE
- Tibialis posterior is the largest of the medial tendons, measuring 4–6 mm in diameter. It may be followed to its insertion into the navicular where the fibres normally fan out.
- Peroneus brevis inserts into the base of the 5th metatarsal. Peroneus longus crosses the sole to insert at the base of the 1st metatarsal and the medial cuneiform.
- The anterior recess may normally contain up to 3 mm depth of fluid. Fluid may normally be identified in the tibialis posterior tendon sheath at or below malleolar level, and within the peroneal tendons below malleolar level and may be asymmetric. The anterior tendons do not normally show surrounding fluid. Flexor digitorum longus and flexor hallucis longus may normally show surrounding fluid on MRI scan, but this is not reported on ultrasound.

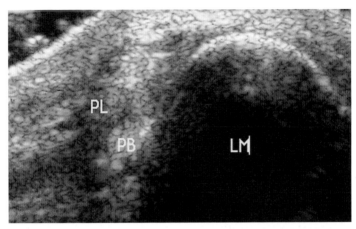

Figure 77a   Transverse plane through the lateral malleolus of the ankle (LM) demonstrating the peroneus longus (PL) and peroneus brevis (PB) tendons

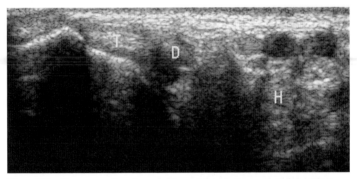

Figure 77b   Transverse plane through the medial ankle demonstrating the tibialis posterior (T), flexor digitorum longus (D) and flexor hallucis longus (H) tendons

FURTHER READING

Hashimoto BE, Kramer DJ, Wiitala L. Applications of musculoskeletal sonography. *Journal of Clinical Ultrasound* 1999;**27**:293–318.

Nazarian LN, Nandkumar MR, Martin CE, Schweitzer ME. Synovial fluid in the hindfoot and ankle: detection of amount and distribution with US. *Radiology* 1995; **197**: 275–278.

Achilles tendon

POSITION
Prone with feet hanging over the edge of the examination couch.

PROBE
7.0–10.0 MHz linear transducer

METHOD
Transducer placed over the Achilles tendon longitudinally and transversely to assess the full length of the tendon from musculotendinous junction to calcaneal insertion. Dorsiflexion of the ankle is helpful to fully evaluate tears.

APPEARANCE
The Achilles tendon has a rounded or C-shape in transverse section. The calcaneal insertion of the tendon may appear low-reflective due to anisotropy or the presence of cartilage at the enthesis. The plantaris tendon should be separately identified as it runs from the posterolateral knee to insert on the posteromedial calcaneus. The retrocalcaneal bursa lies between the Achilles tendon and the calcaneus.

MEASUREMENTS
- Up to 3 mm depth of fluid may normally be identified in the retrocalcaneal bursa.
- Achilles tendon is taken at the level of the medial malleolus in the transverse direction to obtain the anteroposterior measurement: normal: (age range 12–78 years): 5.3 mm (range 4–6 mm)

FURTHER READING
Fornage BD. Achilles tendon: US examination. *Radiology* 1986;**159**:759–764.

Hashimoto BE, Kramer DJ, Wiitala L. Applications of musculoskeletal sonography. *Journal of Clinical Ultrasound* 1999;**27**:293–318.

Nazarian LN, Nandkumar MR, Martin CE, Schweitzer ME. Synovial fluid in the hindfoot and ankle: detection of amount and distribution with US. *Radiology* 1995;**197**:275–278.

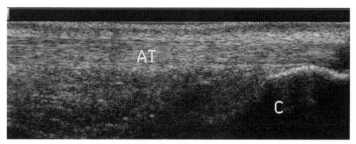

Figure 78 Longitudinal plane through the Achilles tendon (AT) at the insertion into the posterior aspect of the calcaneal bone (C)

LOWER LIMB – FOOT

Plantar fascia

POSITION
Prone with feet hanging over the examination couch.

PROBE
7.0–10.0 MHz linear array transducer.

METHOD
The transducer is placed longitudinally and transversely across the plantar fascia. The origin is at the calcaneal tuberosity, and the fascia is traced to the midarch but becomes superficial and thin in the fore-foot. Measurements of the thickness of the proximal plantar fascia are taken in the longitudinal plane close to the calcaneal attachment.

APPEARANCE
The plantar fascia is well defined and of moderately high reflectivity with a uniform fibrillary pattern, but may be low-reflective at the calcaneal tuberosity due to anisotropy.

	Mean ± SD, (mm)	Range (mm)
Control	3.3 ± 0.38	2.4–4.3
Plantar fasciitis	5.9 ± 0.97	4.1–9.1

FURTHER READING
Gibbon WW, Long G. Ultrasound of plantar aponeurosis (fascia). *Skeletal Radiology* 1999;**28**:21–26.

Hashimoto BE, Kramer DJ, Wiitala L. Applications of musculoskeletal sonography. *Journal of Clinical Ultrasound* 1999;**27**:293–318.

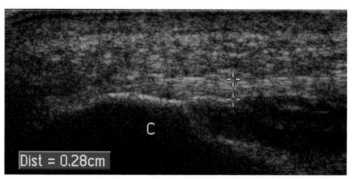

Figure 79 Longitudinal plane through the plantar surface of the foot over the calcaneal bone (C), with the plantar fascia demonstrated between the cursors

Interdigital web spaces

POSITION
Supine

PROBE
7.0–10.0 MHz linear array transducer.

METHOD
The transducer is placed transversely across the dorsum of the foot to examine the spaces between the metatarsal heads. At the same time finger pressure is applied to the plantar surface of web space under examination. Alternatively, forced flexion of the toes, or squeezing of the metatarsal heads together by pressure from the examiner's hand, may displace a neuroma towards the probe for improved visualization. The process is repeated with the probe on the plantar surface and finger pressure on the dorsum of the foot.

APPEARANCE
The normal interspace appears as high-reflective fat bounded by the high-reflective metatarsal cortex on each side. A Morton's neuroma appears as a non-compressible low-reflective mass, whilst a bursa is a compressible low-reflective mass.

FURTHER READING
Redd RA, Peters VJ, Emery SF, Branch HM, Rifkin MD. Morton neuroma: sonographic evaluation. *Radiology* 1989;**171**:415–417.

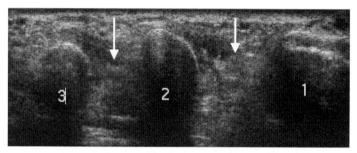

Figure 80 The first (1), second (2) and third (3) metatarsals are visualized on this transverse image at the dorsum of the distal foot, with the interdigital webspaces indicated (arrows) within which a Morton's neuroma may occur

10 PERIPHERAL VASCULAR SYSTEM (ARTERIAL)

Zelena A. Aziz and
Paul S. Sidhu

Upper limbs – peripheral arteries   212
Abdominal aorta and common
    iliac arteries   214
Lower limbs – peripheral arteries   218
Lower limbs – peripheral arteries
    for stenosis   220
Extracranial arteries   222
Extracranial arteries – measurement
    of internal carotid artery stenosis   226
Transcranial Doppler ultrasound   230

Upper limbs – peripheral arteries

PREPARATION
Patient should rest in a supine position for 15 minutes in a room where temperature is 21°C to avoid vasoconstriction.

POSITION
Supine.

PROBE
5–7.5 MHz linear transducer.

METHOD
Examination of the upper extremity usually starts at the level of the subclavian artery followed by the axillary artery, brachial artery and the radial and ulnar arteries. The radial and ulnar arteries are imaged with the arm in supination, and slightly abducted. The vessels should be examined in the longitudinal axis.

APPEARANCE
The arteries appear as non-compressible, pulsating tubular structures. Due to their high peripheral resistance the spectral Doppler waveform arising from peripheral arteries show a typical triphasic flow pattern, consisting of a steep systolic upslope, a systolic peak, a reverse flow component, forward flow in late diastole and presystolic zero.

MEASUREMENTS

Artery	Diameter (mean ± SD, mm)	Flow velocity (mean ± SD, cm/s)
Subclavian	–	100 ± 49
Brachial	3.5 ± 0.9	75 ± 18
Radial (wrist)	2.8 ± 0.6	57 ± 16
Ulnar (wrist)	2.8 ± 0.6	66 ± 27

FURTHER READING
Trager S, Pignataro M, Anderson J, Kleinert JM. Color flow Doppler: imaging the upper extremity. *Journal of Hand Surgery (Am)* 1993;**18**:621–625.

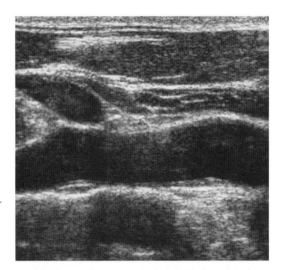

Figure 81a The subclavian artery is visualized in a longitudinal plane by placing the linear probe in the supraclavicular fossa and angling caudally

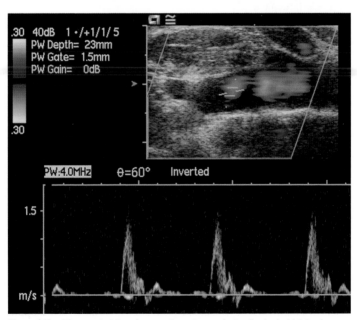

Figure 81b The spectral Doppler waveform demonstrates the typical triphasic waveform pattern

Abdominal aorta and common iliac arteries

PREPARATION
None.

POSITION
Examine in the supine position. Left anterior oblique as needed.

PROBE
1.5–5 MHz curvilinear transducer.

APPEARANCE
Pulsating tubular low-reflective structure lying slightly to the left of the midline, anterior to the vertebral column. The distal aorta is most often involved in aneurysmal dilatations. An enlargement of the distal aorta and common iliac artery should be considered when:

- The luminal diameter exceeds 23 mm in the distal aorta and 14 mm in the common iliac artery in men, and 19 mm and 12 mm respectively in women.
- There is demonstration of focal enlargement.

METHOD
Arms along the body to relax the abdominal wall. Luminal size of the abdominal aorta can be measured at two levels;

- *Proximal diameter:* At the level of the confluence of the splenic and portal veins and the left renal vein.
- *Distal diameter:* Measure just above aortic bifurcation.
- *Luminal diameter of the common iliac artery:* Measure just distal to the aortic bifurcation. Anteroposterior diameter is measured in both transverse and longitudinal sections from inner edge of the anterior wall to the inner edge of the posterior wall.

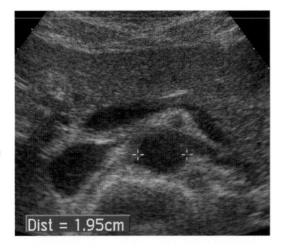

Figure 82a
Measurement at the confluence of the splenic and portal veins at the level of the left renal vein; the proximal diameter

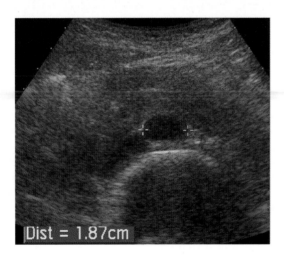

Figure 82b
Measurement just above the aortic bifurcation; the distal diameter

MEASUREMENTS

	Age (years)		Vessel diameter (mean ± SD, mm)	Range (mm)
Proximal aorta	15–49	Male	16.9 ± 2.4	12–22
		Female	15.0 ± 2.4	11–22
	50–89	Male	19.9 ± 3.4	14–28
		Female	18.3 ± 2.7	14–25
Distal aorta	15–49	Male	15.1 ± 1.7	12–19
		Female	12.7 ± 1.3	10–16
	50–89	Male	16.8 ± 2.9	11–23
		Female	14.6 ± 1.9	11–18
Common iliac artery	15–49	Male	9.7 ± 1.2	7.5–11.5
		Female	8.5 ± 1.0	6–10
	50–89	Male	10.1 ± 2.0	6.5–16.5
		Female	9.2 ± 1.3	7–13

FURTHER READING

Pedersen OM, Aslaksen A, Vik-Mo H. Ultrasound measurement of the luminal diameter of the abdominal aorta and iliac arteries in patients without vascular disease. *Journal of Vascular Surgery* 1993;**17**:596–601.

Lower limbs – peripheral arteries

PREPARATION
Patient should rest in a supine position for 15 minutes in a room where temperature is 21°C to avoid vasoconstriction.

POSITION
Supine. For the popliteal region and lower leg the patient should be moved to a later decubitus position or the prone position.

PROBE
5–7.5 MHz linear transducer.

METHOD
Major arteries should be imaged in the longitudinal plane. Color Doppler imaging is performed from the midaspect of the artery under investigation and the Doppler angle kept at <60°.

APPEARANCE
The arteries appear as non-compressible, pulsating tubular structures. If calcified, color and spectral Doppler interrogation is difficult. Due to the high peripheral resistance the spectral Doppler waveform arising from peripheral arteries show a typical triphasic flow pattern, consisting of a steep systolic up-slope, a systolic peak, a reverse flow component, forward flow in late diastole and presystolic zero.

MEASUREMENTS

Arterial segment	Peak systolic velocity (mean ± SD, cm/s)
Distal common iliac	90 ± 21
Distal common femoral	71 ± 15
Profunda femoris	64 ± 15
Proximal superficial femoral	73 ± 10
Mid superficial femoral	74 ± 13
Distal superficial femoral	56 ± 12
Distal popliteal	53 ± 4
Tibioperoneal trunk	57 ± 14
Proximal anterior tibial	40 ± 7
Proximal posterior tibial	42 ± 14
Proximal peroneal	46 ± 14

Figure 83a
Longitudinal plane through the proximal superficial femoral artery, above the superficial femoral vein (arrow)

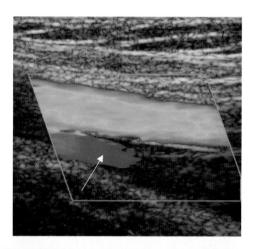

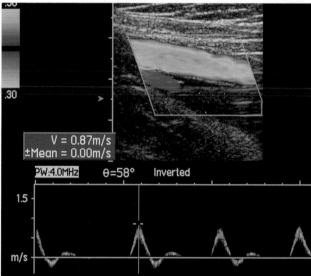

Figure 83b Normal spectral Doppler waveform pattern through the superficial femoral artery demonstrating a normal triphasic waveform pattern

FURTHER READING
Hatsukami TS, Primozich J, Zierler RE, Strandness DE Jr: Color Doppler characteristics in normal lower extremity arteries. *Ultrasound in Medicine and Biology* 1992; **18**:167–171.

Lower limbs – peripheral arteries for stenosis

PREPARATION
Patient should rest in a supine position for 15 minutes in a room where temperature is 21°C to avoid vasoconstriction.

POSITION
Supine. For examination of the popliteal region and lower leg the patient should be moved to a lateral decubitus position or the prone position.

PROBE
5–7.5 MHz linear transducer.

METHOD
Major arteries should be imaged in the longitudinal plane. Color Doppler imaging is performed from the midaspect of the artery under investigation and the Doppler angle kept at <60°. The normal presystolic velocity (PSV_n) is measured in a normal segment of artery proximal to the stenosis, and the stenotic presystolic velocity (PSV_s) is measured at the region of highest color turbulence to indicate the area of maximum velocity, and therefore greatest stenosis.

APPEARANCE
The arteries appear as non-compressible, pulsating tubular structures. If calcified, Doppler interrogation is difficult. Plaque appears as intraluminal areas of varying reflectivity.

MEASUREMENTS

% Stenosis	PSV (cm/s)	PSV_s/PSV_n
>50	120	1.4
>70	160	2.0
>90	180	2.9

FURTHER READING
Sacks D, Robinson ML, Marinelli DL, Perlmutter GS. *Journal of Ultrasound in Medicine* 1992;**11**:95–103.

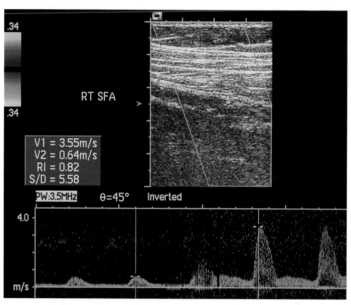

Figure 84   The spectral Doppler gate has been moved from the proximal superficial femoral artery to a point just distal to a focal stenosis. The peak systolic velocity measured before the stenosis is 64 cm/s and distal to the stenosis 355 cm/s, indicating a stenosis of more than 90% (Courtesy of Dr Colin R. Deane)

Extracranial arteries

PREPARATION
None.

POSITION
Supine. Neck extended and head turned slightly away from the side being examined.

PROBE
5.0–8.0 MHz linear transducer.

METHOD
Examine the common carotid artery (CCA), internal carotid artery (ICA), external carotid artery (ECA) and vertebral arteries in transverse and longitudinal planes. The ICA runs lateral or posterolateral to the ECA in its first part and the extracranial portion does not give off any branches.

APPEARANCE
Waveforms: The spectral Doppler waveform of the ICA is low resistance with a high diastolic component in comparison to the ECA, which is of high resistance with a low diastolic component. The waveform of the CCA is usually of low resistance, but may appear as a hybrid of those of the ICA and ECA. The waveform of the vertebral artery is of low resistance similar to that of the ICA but with lower amplitude.

Plaque morphology: Plaque disease not causing significant arterial narrowing but with features such as haemorrhage and ulceration may be associated with cerebrovascular symptoms. Plaque morphology has been classified into categories:

- *Types 1–4*, with Type 1 being low-reflective and Type 4 being uniformly high-reflective. Type 2 and 3 are intermediate forms. Low-reflective areas seen on ultrasound of an atherosclerotic plaque imply a greater risk of symptomatic cerebrovascular disease, although controversy exists as to the components that make up these low-reflective areas. It has been suggested that fibrous plaques are high-reflective and stable whereas more low-reflective plaques contain increased lipid and cholesterol levels, which render these plaques unstable. Other studies have suggested that the low-reflective areas of a plaque correlate with areas of intraplaque haemorrhage and are associated with an increased risk of cerebrovascular events.

- *Heterogenous or homogenous*, where heterogenous plaques are those exhibiting major differences in reflectivity. These plaques are the predominant type of plaque in symptomatic patients with a greater than 70% stenosis.
- *Intima-media thickness (IMT):* The inner high-reflective line represents the luminal-intima interface and the outer high-reflective line represents the media-adventitia interface, with the distance between the two lines being a measure of the thickness of the intima and media combined. Measurements should ideally be taken at several sites and averaged as the mean of the maximum IMT in the CCA and ICA. The median wall thickness in adults ranges from between 0.5 mm and 1.0 mm with the measurement increasing with age. Values of 1.0 mm or greater are usually taken to be abnormal.

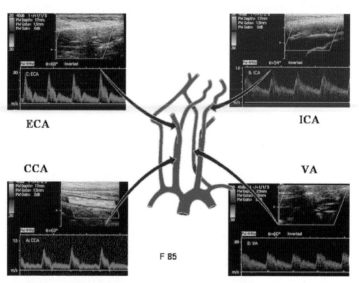

Figure 85 The spectral Doppler waveforms obtained in each of the four sites of measurement in the extracranial carotid arterial system. CCA, common carotid artery; ICA, internal carotid artery; ECA, external carotid artery; VA, vertebral artery

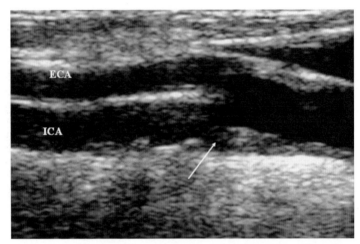

Figure 86a Longitudinal plane through the carotid bifurcation demonstrating the external carotid artery (ECA) and the internal carotid artery (ICA). The arrow points to an ulcerated plaque situated on the posterior wall of the carotid bulb

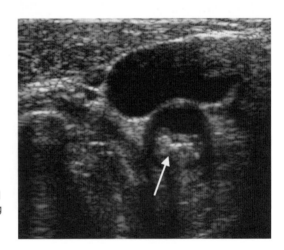

Figure 86b
Transverse plane through the carotid bulb demonstrating a heterogeneous plaque (arrow)

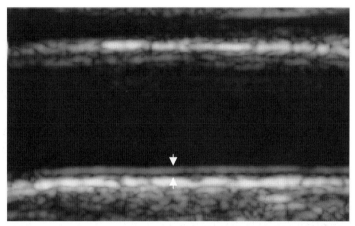

Figure 87 Measurement of the intimal medial thickness is from the inner high-reflective line to the outer high-reflective line (arrows) on the far wall of the common carotid artery close to the carotid bulb

FURTHER READING

Sidhu PS, Allan PL. The extended role of carotid artery ultrasound. *Clinical Radiology* 1997;**52**:643–653.

Sidhu PS, Desai SR. A simple and reproducible method of assessing intimal-medial thickness of the common carotid artery. *British Journal of Radiology* 1997;**70**:85–89.

Steffen CM, Gray-Weale AC, Byrne KE, Lusby RJ. Carotid atheroma ultrasound appearance in symptomatic and asymptomatic vessels. *Australian and New Zealand Journal of Surgery* 1989;**59**:529–534.

Extracranial arteries – measurement of internal carotid artery stenosis

PREPARATION
None.

POSITION
Supine. Neck extended and head turned slightly away from the side being examined.

PROBE
5.0–8.0 MHz linear transducer.

METHOD
Examine the common carotid artery (CCA), internal carotid artery (ICA), external carotid artery (ECA) and vertebral arteries in transverse and longitudinal planes. The ICA runs lateral or posterolateral to the ECA in its first part and the extracranial portion does not give off any branches.

APPEARANCES
Grayscale imaging by direct measurement of luminal reduction; measurement of luminal diameter and area reduction should be made on the cross-section of the vessel. Spectral Doppler analysis; many parameters have been suggested to quantify a 70% diameter reduction, and different centres will have their own established diagnostic criteria. The establishment of spectral Doppler criteria for grading clinically significant carotid stenosis of 70% or more is the objective in assessment of internal carotid artery (ICA) stenosis, as symptomatic patients benefit from carotid endarterectomy.

MEASUREMENTS
Velocity measurements are most easily obtained on longitudinal images away from the bifurcation. Flow velocity must be angle corrected and a standard examination angle, as near as possible to 60° should be used. The two velocity parameters commonly used are the peak systolic velocity (PSV) and the ratio of the PSV at the maximal ICA stenosis to the PSV in the normal ipsilateral common carotid artery (CCA). The end diastolic velocity (EDV) may be used as a discriminator at higher of stenosis. 'String-flow' occurs when the stenosis is severe enough (>95%) to cause a drop in velocity.

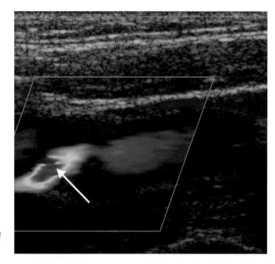

Figure 88a An area of high-color turbulence (arrow) is detected in the proximal internal carotid artery indicating an area of arterial narrowing

Diameter reduction (%)	PSV (cm/s)	EDV (cm/s)	PSV_{ICA}/PSV_{CCA}
0–29	<100	<40	<3.2
30–49	110–130	<40	<3.2
50–59	>130	<40	<3.2
60–69	>130	40–110	3.2–4.0
70–79	>230	110–140	>4.0
80–95	>230	>140	>4.0

FURTHER READING

Grant EG, Benson CB, Moneta GL *et al*. Carotid artery stenosis: gray-scale and Doppler US diagnosis. Society of Radiologists in Ultrasound Consensus Conference. *Radiology* 2003;**229**:350–346.

Moneta GL, Edwards JM, Papanicolaou G, Hatsukami T, Taylor LM, Strandess DE, Porter JM. Screening for asymptomatic internal carotid artery stenosis: duplex criteria for discriminating 60% to 99% stenosis. *Journal of Vascular Surgery* 1992;**21**:989–994.

Moneta GL, Edwards JM, Chitwood RW, Taylor LM, Cummings CA, Porter JM. Correlation of North American Symptomatic Carotid Endarterectomy Trial (NASCET) angiographic definition of 70% to 99% internal carotid stenosis with duplex scanning. *Journal of Vascular Surgery* 1993;**17**:152–159.

Sidhu PS, Allan PL. Ultrasound assessment of internal carotid artery stenosis. *Clinical Radiology* 1997;**52**:654–658.

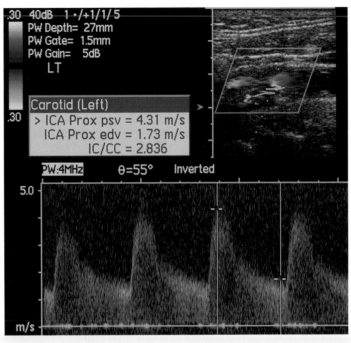

Figure 88b A spectral Doppler gate is placed over the area of color turbulence and a peak systolic velocity of 4.31 m/s and an end diastolic velocity of 1.73 m/s is obtained, suggesting a stenosis of 80–95%

Transcranial Doppler ultrasound

PREPARATION
None.

POSITION
Patient supine and facing forward for the transtemporal and transorbital views and sitting with the head flexed forward for the transforaminal view.

PROBE
2.0–2.5 MHz curvilinear transducer with a small footprint.

METHOD
Transtemporal approach: The suprasellar cistern or midbrain is identified and used to locate the circle of Willis. The ipsilateral anterior, middle and posterior cerebral arteries can be identified; the posterior communicating arteries are difficult to locate. The contralateral arteries may be seen. The terminal internal carotid artery may be seen in the coronal plane.

Transforaminal approach: Identify the vertebral arteries and follow anteriorly and superiorly to identify the basilar artery.

Transorbital approach: Transducer face placed on the closed eyelid, directed through the orbit to identify the ipsilateral internal carotid and ophthalmic arteries.

APPEARANCES
Using color Doppler will enable the arteries to be located and aid in the placement of the spectral Doppler gate to measure arterial velocity. Power output should be reduced for the transorbital views. The spectral Doppler waveforms will reflect the low resistance of the intracranial arteries, with a broad systolic peak and high forward diastolic flow; a low resistance index (RI) will be documented.

Figure 89a The transcranial ultrasound probe is placed over the right temporal bone, and following an infusion of microbubble ultrasound contrast, the intracranial arteries are clearly depicted. MCA R; right middle cerebral artery; P1 PCA R; first portion of the right posterior cerebral artery; P1 PCA L; first part of the left posterior cerebral artery; A1

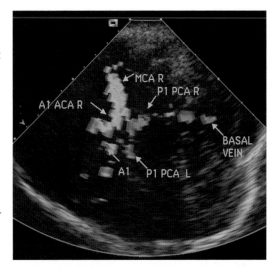

ACA R; first part of the right anterior cerebral artery; A1 first part of the left anterior cerebral artery

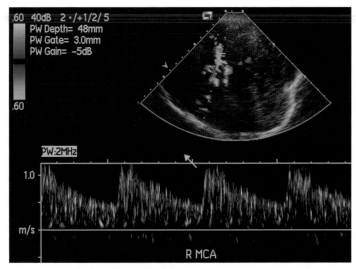

Figure 89b A spectral Doppler gate is placed over the right middle cerebral artery (R MCA) to obtain a normal low-resistance spectral Doppler waveform pattern

MEASUREMENTS

Flow velocities and RI (mean ± 95%CI)[1]

	Age (years)		
	20–39	40–59	>60
Anterior cerebral artery			
PSV	91 (87–95)	88 (83–93)	79 (75–84)
EDV	41 (39–43)	42 (40–45)	33 (31–35)
RI	0.53 (0.52–0.55)	0.53 (0.51–0.54)	0.59 (0.57–0.62)
Middle cerebral artery			
PSV	113 (109–116)	106 (101–111)	92 (88–96)
EDV	51 (49–53)	47 (45–50)	35 (33–37)
RI	0.55 (0.53–0.56)	0.54 (0.54–0.56)	0.62 (0.60–0.64)
Posterior cerebral artery			
PSV	81 (78–84)	71 (68–74)	66 (63–69)
EDV	36 (35–38)	33 (31–35)	26 (24–28)
RI	0.54 (0.53–0.56)	0.53 (0.52–0.55)	0.60 (0.58–0.62)
Vertebral artery			
PSV	66 (63–69)	59 (55–63)	52 (48–55)
EDV	31 (29–32)	27 (26–29)	22 (20–24)
RI	0.54 (0.53–0.56)	0.53 (0.51–0.54)	0.59 (0.57–0.61)
Basilar artery			
PSV	74 (70–78)	63 (56–69)	54 (49–59)
EDV	34 (32–36)	29 (26–32)	23 (20–26)
RI	0.51 (0.46–0.56)	0.53 (0.51–0.55)	0.60 (0.56–0.64)

PSV, peak systolic velocity (cm/s); EDV, end diastolic velocity (cm/s); RI, resistance index.

REFERENCE
1. Martin PJ, Evans DH, Naylor AR. Transcranial color-coded sonography of the basal cerebral circulation. Reference data from 115 volunteers. *Stroke* 1994;**25**:390–396.

FURTHER READING
Lupetin AR, Davis DA, Beckman I, Dash N. Transcranial Doppler. Part 1. Principles, technique, and normal appearances. *Radiographics* 1995;**15**:179–191.

Ringelstein EB, Kahlscheuer B, Niggemeyer E, Otis SM. Transcranial Doppler sonography: anatomical landmarks and normal velocity measurements. *Ultrasound in Medicine and Biology* 1990;**16**:745–761.

11

PERIPHERAL VASCULAR SYSTEM (VENOUS)

Paul S. Sidhu

Inferior vena cava   236
Neck veins   238
Leg veins   240

Inferior vena cava

PREPARATION
None.

POSITION
Supine.

PROBE
3.5–5.0 MHz curvilinear transducer.

METHOD
The patient is examined in three phases: (1) quiet respiration, (2) during breath holding (Valsalva maneuver) and (3) on leg raising. Examine in the transverse plane in the epigastrium, measure the short and long axis diameter 1 cm below the level of the left renal vein.

APPEARANCE
A tubular structure lying to the right of the midline, with variable diameter with respiratory cycle.

MEASUREMENTS

Phase	IVC diameter (mm)	
	Mean	Range
Quiet respiration	17.2	5.1–28.9
Breath holding	18.8	7.7–31.3
Leg raising	17.6	9.7–31.0

FURTHER READING
Sykes AM, McLoughlin RF, So CBB, Cooperberg PL, Mathieson JR, Gray RR, Brandt R. Sonographic assessment of infrarenal inferior vena caval dimensions. *Journal of Ultrasound in Medicine* 1995;**14**:665–668.

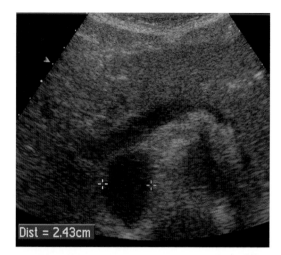

Figure 90a
Transverse plane through the epigastrium measuring the diameter of the inferior vena cava during quiet respiration

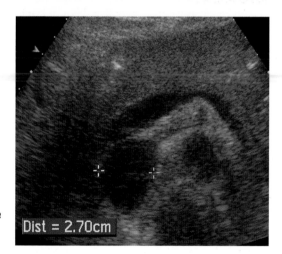

Figure 90b
Measurement at the same level during breath holding

Neck veins

PREPARATION
None.

POSITION
Supine.

PROBE
5.0–8.0 MHz linear transducer.

METHOD
Both longitudinal and transverse planes to examine the vessels. Spectral Doppler measurements are made in the longitudinal plane, with angle correction applied.

APPEARANCE
The vessel lumen is echo-free, the veins are compressible and the venous confluence is Y-shaped. Blood flow is symmetrical and biphasic in 57%, continuous and monophasic in 29% and monophasic in 13%. Velocity is less than 100 cm/s.

MEASUREMENTS

Measurement location	End systolic velocity (mean ± SD, cm/s)[1]
Right internal jugular	28 ± 15
Right innominate	33 ± 16
Right subclavian	16 ± 10
Left internal jugular	22 ± 16
Left innominate	22 ± 11
Left subclavian	11 ± 7

REFERENCE
1. Pucheu A, Evans J, Thomas D, Scheuble C, Pucheu M. Doppler ultrasonography of normal neck veins. *Journal of Clinical Ultrasound* 1994;**22**:367–373.

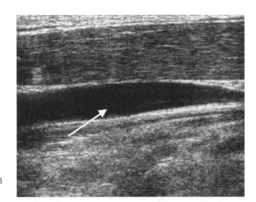

Figure 91a
Longitudinal plane
demonstrating the
internal jugular vein
(arrow)

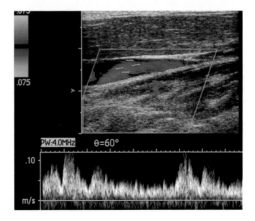

Figure 91b
Transverse plane
through the internal
jugular vein (arrow)
adjacent to the
common carotid
artery

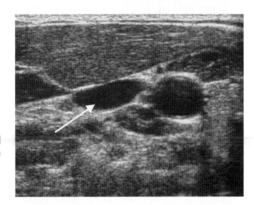

Figure 91c
Spectral Doppler
waveform obtained
from the internal
jugular vein
demonstrating a
normal spectral
waveform pattern

Leg veins

PREPARATION
None.

POSITION
Supine.

PROBE
4.0–6.0 MHz linear array transducer.

METHOD
Measurements performed at the common femoral vein, high superficial vein, mid superficial femoral vein, low superficial femoral vein and the popliteal vein. Anteroposterior measurements taken in the transverse plane. A vein-to-artery ratio can be calculated from an arterial measurement at the same level as the vein measurement. Veins with an acute thrombosis are larger and veins with a chronic thrombosis are smaller than normal veins. There is considerable overlap in the measurements.

APPEARANCE
The veins of the legs are identified as echo-poor structures that are readily compressible, with a continuous forward spectral Doppler trace with some respiratory modulation.

MEASUREMENTS
Vein-to-artery ratio calculated by dividing the anteroposterior vein diameter by the anteroposterior artery diameter at the same point.

Vessel	Vein diameter (mean ± SD, mm)	Vein/artery ratio (mean ± SD)
Common femoral vein	10.57 ± 2.88	1.34 ± 0.37
High superficial vein	7.10 ± 1.96	1.24 ± 0.36
Mid superficial vein	6.41 ± 1.72	1.21 ± 0.33
Low superficial vein	6.52 ± 1.74	1.19 ± 0.32
Popliteal vein	6.80 ± 2.11	1.22 ± 0.36

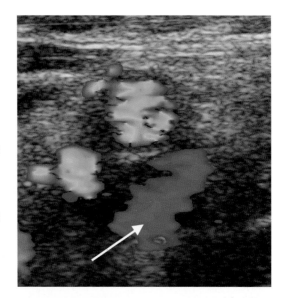

Figure 92a Color Doppler flow is seen in the superficial femoral vein (arrow) in the transverse plane at the level of the bifurcation of the superficial femoral artery and deep femoral artery

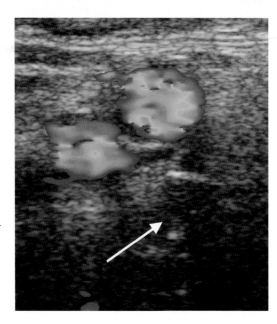

Figure 92b Compression completely obliterates the color Doppler flow and lumen of the superficial femoral vein; there is no intraluminal thrombus

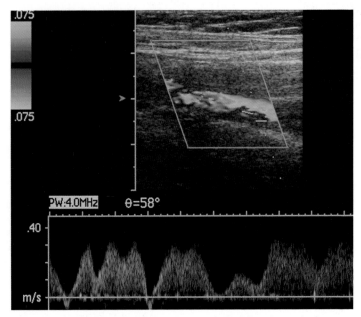

Figure 92c Spectral Doppler waveform pattern obtained from the proximal aspect of the superficial femoral vein showing a normal configuration

FURTHER READING

Hertzberg BS, Kliewer MA, DeLong DM, Lalouche KJ, Paulson EK, Frederick MG, Carroll BA. Sonographic assessment of lower limb vein diameters: implications for the diagnosis and characterization of deep venous thrombosis. *American Journal of Roentgenology* 1997;**168**:1253–1257.

12 OBSTETRICS

Wui K. Chong,
Anthony E. Swartz and
Janice Newsome

Comparison of serum β-hCG
levels and ultrasound
landmarks to gestational
age on transvaginal
sonography (first trimester) 244

Gestational sac (first
trimester) 246

Fetal heartbeat (first
trimester) 250

Crown–rump length 252

Nuchal fold thickness 254

Nuchal translucency
thickness 256

Biparietal diameter 258

Head circumference 262

Abdominal circumference 266

Multiple fetal parameters in
the assessment of
gestational age 270

Ratio of head to abdomen
circumference 274

Estimated fetal weight
based on biparietal
diameter and abdominal
circumference 276

Fetal femur length 286

Fetal humerus length 290

Systolic/diastolic ratio in
the umbilical artery 294

Cerebral ventricles – lateral
ventricle transverse atrial
measurement 298

Cisterna magna 300

Thoracic circumference 302

Renal pelvis diameter 304

Mean renal lengths for
gestational ages 306

Outer orbital diameter 308

Fetal stomach diameter 312

Fetal small bowel 314

Fetal colon 316

Predicted fetal weight
percentiles throughout
pregnancy 318

Amniotic fluid 320

Comparison of serum β-hCG levels and ultrasound landmarks to gestational age on transvaginal sonography (first trimester)

PREPARATION
Empty bladder for transvaginal imaging

POSITION
Midsagittal image through embryo

PROBE
Transvaginal: 5.0- 8.0 MHz transducer

METHOD
Longest dimension of embryo from top of skull to bottom of torso. The extremities are not included.

APPEARANCE
Embryo: Figure-of-eight shaped solid structure within gestational sac.
Gestational sac: Fluid collection with high-reflective rim embedded within the endometrium.
Yolk sac: Spherical cystic structure with well-defined high-reflective margin lying within gestational sac.

MEASUREMENTS

β-hCG[a] (mIU/ml)	Ultrasound landmarks	Gestational age (days)
1000	Gestational sac	32
7200	Yolk sac	36–40
10 000	Embryo with heart motion	40

[a] First International Reference Preparation.

Other predictors of abnormal outcome:
• Mean sac diameter (MSD) – crown–rump length (CRL) <5 mm (valid up to 9 weeks gestational age)
• Yolk sac >5.6 mm (5–10 weeks gestational age).

FURTHER READING

Bree RL, Edwards M, Bohm-Velez M, Beyler S, Roberts J, Mendelson EB. Transvaginal sonography in the evaluation of normal early pregnancy: Correlation with HCG level. *American Journal of Roentgenology* 1989;**153**:75–79.

Keith SC, London SN, Weitzman GA, O'Brien TJ, Miller MM. Serial transvaginal ultrasound scans and beta-human chorionic gonadotrophin levels in early singleton and multiple pregnancies. *Fertility and Sterility* 1993;**59**:1007–1010.

Gestational sac (first trimester)

PREPARATION
Empty bladder.

POSITION
Supine. Sagittal and transverse images of the endometrial stripe.

PROBE
5.0–8.0 MHz transvaginal transducer is used for early first-trimester imaging.

METHOD

$$\text{mean sac diameter (MSD)} = \frac{\text{sum of three right orthogonal measurements}}{3}$$

APPEARANCE
Gestational sac is normally visualized by 4.5 weeks with transvaginal sonography (TVS) as a small fluid collection with high-reflective rim embedded within the endometrium.

MEASUREMENTS
β-hCG threshold level above which gestational sac should be seen on TVS:
- singleton 1000 mIU/ml (First International Reference Preparation)
- twin 1556 mIU/ml
- IVF/GIFT 3372 mIU/ml

Yolk sac normally visible (TVS)[1] if MSD >8 mm
Embryo normally visible (TVS)[1] if MSD >16 mm
Nonvisualization above these threshold levels is suggestive of non-viable pregnancy.[1]

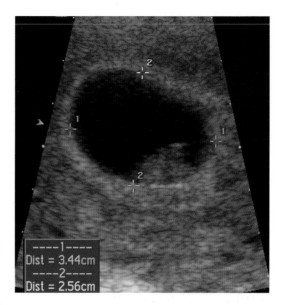

Figure 93 The gestational sac is identified as a fluid collection (cursors) with an embryo present (Courtesy of Jane L. Clarke)

Mean sac diameter (mm)	Estimates of gestational age[1]	
	Mean (weeks)	95%CI (days)
2	5.0	34.9 (34.3–35.5)
3	5.1	35.8 (35.2–36.3)
4	5.2	36.6 (36.1–37.2)
5	5.4	37.5 (37.0–38.0)
6	5.5	38.4 (37.9–38.9)
7	5.6	39.3 (38.9–39.7)
8	5.7	40.2 (39.8–40.6)
9	5.9	41.1 (40.7–41.4)
10	6.0	41.9 (41.6–42.3)
11	6.1	42.8 (42.5–43.2)
12	6.2	43.7 (43.4–44.0)
13	6.4	44.6 (44.3–44.9)
14	6.5	45.5 (45.2–45.8)
15	6.6	46.3 (46.0–46.6)
16	6.7	47.2 (46.9–47.5)
17	6.9	48.1 (47.8–48.4)
18	7.0	49.0 (48.6–49.4)
20	7.3	50.8 (50.3–51.2)
22	7.5	52.5 (52.0–53.0)
25	7.9	55.2 (54.6–55.7)
30	8.5	59.6 (58.8–60.4)

REFERENCE
1. Daya S, Woods S, Ward S, Lappalainen R, Caco C: Early pregnancy assessment with transvaginal ultrasound scanning. *Canadian Medical Association Journal* 1991;15:441–446.

Fetal heartbeat (first trimester)

PREPARATION
Empty bladder for transvaginal imaging.

POSITION
Coronal or sagittal image through embryo. Locate pulsating heart within the embryo.

PROBE
Transvaginal: 5.0–8.0 MHz transducer.

METHOD
M-Mode or spectral Doppler gate placed over pulsating heart. Spectral Doppler should be used sparingly and avoided where possible because it uses greater energy.

APPEARANCE
Fetal heartbeat should be visible if the crown–rump length (CRL) is 5 mm or greater on transvaginal sonography.[1]

MEASUREMENTS
Fetal bradycardia.

CRL (mm)	Heart rate (beats/min)[2]
<5	<80
5–9	<100
10–15	<110

REFERENCES
1. Laing FC. Ultrasound evaluation during the first trimester of pregnancy. In: Callen PW. *Ultrasonography in Obstetrics and Gynaecology*, 4th edn, WB Saunders, Philadelphia, 2000.
2. Howe RS, Isaacson KJ, Albert JL, Coutifaris CB. Embryonic heart rate in human pregnancy. *Journal of Ultrasound in Medicine* 1991;**10**:367–371.

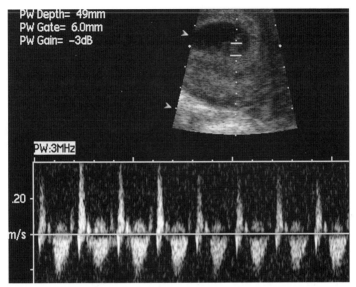

Figure 94 A spectral Doppler gate is placed over the embryo, which has a crown–rump length of more than 5 mm, to demonstrate the normal fetal heartbeat (Courtesy of Jane L. Clarke)

Crown–rump length

PREPARATION
Empty bladder for transvaginal imaging. Full bladder for trans-abdominal imaging in first trimester.

POSITION
Midsagittal image through embryo. Midcoronal plane less accurate because flexion/extension cannot be determined and should only be used as last resort.

PROBE
Transabdominal: 3.0–5.0 MHz curvilinear transducer
Transvaginal: 5.0–8.0 MHz transducer

METHOD
Accurate only in first trimester. Longest dimension of embryo from top of skull to bottom of torso. The extremities are not included. Embryo should not be flexed.

APPEARANCE
Bilobed solid density within gestational sac. Spine should be visible in long axis in midsagittal view in late first trimester.

MEASUREMENTS
Predicted menstrual age (MA, weeks) from CRL measurements (mm) from 5.7 to 12 weeks[1] (95%CI is ± 8% of the predicted age)

CRL (mm)	MA (wks)	CRL (mm)	MA (wks)	CRL (mm)	MA (wks)
2	5.7	12	7.4	31	10.0
3	5.9	14	7.7	33	10.2
4	6.1	16	8.0	35	10.4
5	6.2	18	8.3	37	10.6
6	6.4	20	8.6	40	10.9
7	6.6	22	8.9	43	11.2
8	6.7	24	9.1	46	11.4
9	6.9	26	9.4	49	11.7
10	7.1	28	9.6	53	12.0

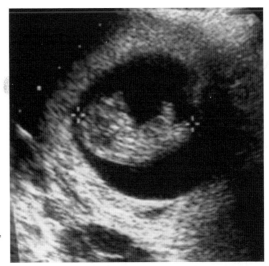

Figure 95
Crown–rump length (between cursors) is obtained by positioning the cursors from the apex of the skull to the base of the torso, not including the limbs

REFERENCE

1. Hadlock FP, Shah YP, Kanon DJ, Math B, Lindsey JV. Fetal crown-rump length: Re-evaluation of relation to menstrual age (5–18 weeks) with high-resolution real-time US. *Radiology* 1992;**182**:501–505.

Nuchal fold thickness

PREPARATION
Full bladder for transabdominal imaging.

POSITION
Axial plane through fetal skull angled posteriorly to include cerebellum.

PROBE
3.0–5.0 MHz transducer is used for all second- and third-trimester obstetric imaging.

METHOD
Performed between 14 and 21 weeks gestation. Maximum distance from the outer skull table to the outer skin edge. The cerebellum should be symmetrical with the cavum septum pellucidum visualized anteriorly.

APPEARANCE
Thickening of soft tissue of the neck posterior to the occiput.

MEASUREMENTS
Normal: ≤5 mm between 14–18 weeks increases with gestational age. Nuchal fold thickness ≥6 mm between 14–18 weeks is suggestive of Down's syndrome

FURTHER READING
Benacerraf BR, Barss VA, Laboda LA. A sonographic sign for the detection in the second trimester of the fetus with Down's syndrome. *American Journal of Obstetrics and Gynecology* 1985;**151**:1078–1079.

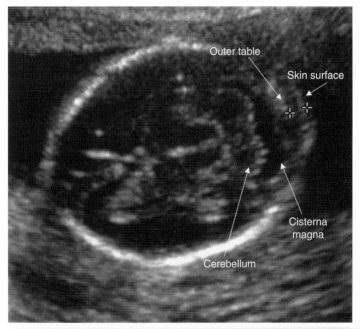

Figure 96   Nuchal fold thickness is measured from the outer table of the skull to the skin surface at the level of the cerebellum in the axial plane (between cursors)

Nuchal translucency thickness

PREPARATION
Full bladder for transabdominal imaging

POSITION
Midsagittal image through embryo.

PROBE
- *Transabdominal*: 3.0–5.0 MHz transducer
- *Transvaginal*: 5–8Mhz transducer.

METHOD
Performed at 11–14 weeks. Thickness of the cystic area posterior to the occiput *alone* is measured. The skin surface and occiput are excluded. Calipers on machine should be capable of measuring down to 0.1 mm.

APPEARANCE
Cystic area in the soft tissue posterior to the occiput.

MEASUREMENTS
Normal nuchal translucency (NT) increases with gestational age:
- 95th centile NT thickness at crown-rump length of 38 mm = 2.2 mm
- 95th centile NT thickness at crown-rump length of 84 mm = 2.8 mm

Increased NT thickness is suggestive of chromosomal disorders (especially trisomy 21, cystic hygroma and skeletal dysplasias). Cutoff figures of 2.5 mm, 3 mm and 95th centile have been used.

FURTHER READING

Nicolaides KH, Brizot Ml, Snidjers RJM: Fetal nuchal translucency: ultrasound screening for fetal trisomy in the first trimester of pregnancy. *British Journal of Obstetrics and Gynaecology* 1994;**101**:782–786.

Pajkrt E, van Lith JMM, Mol BWJ, Bleker,OP, Bilardo CM. Screening for Down's syndrome by fetal nuchal translucency measurement in a general obstetric population *Ultrasound in Obstetrics and Gynecology* 1998;**12**:163–169.

Pandya PP, Brizot M, Snidjers RJM, Nicolaides KH First Trimester fetal nuchal translucency thickness and risk for trisomies. *Obstetrics and Gynecology* 1994;**84**:420–423.

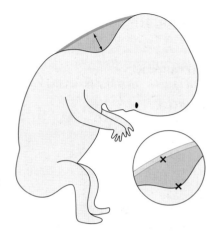

Figure 97 Thickness of the cystic area posterior to the occiput alone is measured, carefully excluding the skin surface and occiput

Biparietal diameter

PREPARATION
Full bladder for transabdominal imaging in first and second trimester.

POSITION
Transaxial image of fetal skull at level of thalami and cavum septum pellucidum. Transducer must be perpendicular to the parietal bones.

PROBE
3.0–5.0 MHz transducer is used for all second- and third-trimester obstetric imaging.

METHOD
Measured from outer edge of cranium nearest to the transducer to the inner edge of cranium farthest from transducer.

APPEARANCE
Thalami appear as symmetric low-reflective structures on either side of linear midline high-reflective line (third ventricle). Calvaria must appear smooth and symmetric bilaterally.

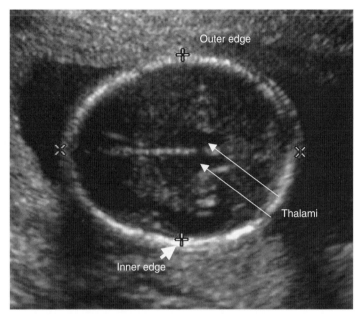

Figure 98   Measurement is taken from the outer edge of the cranium nearest the transducer to inner edge of the cranium furthest from the transducer at the level of the paired thalami (between cursors + and +). The occipitofrontal diameter is measured at the same level (between cursors × and ×)

MEASUREMENTS

Biparietal diameter (mm)	Gestational age (weeks, mean[a] and range[b])	Biparietal diameter (mm)	Gestational age (weeks, mean[a] and range[b])
20	12.0 (12.0	42	18.1 (16.6–19.8)
21	12.0 (12.0)	43	18.4 (16.8–20.2)
22	12.7 (12.2–13.2)	44	18.8 (16.9–20.7)
23	13.0 (12.4–13.6)	45	19.1 (17.0–21.2)
24	13.2 (12.6–13.8)	46	19.4 (17.4–21.4)
25	13.5 (12.9–14.1)	47	19.7 (17.8–21.6)
26	13.7 (13.1–14.3)	48	20.0 (18.2–21.8)
27	14.0 (13.4–14.6)	49	20.3 (18.6–22.0)
28	14.3 (13.6–15.0)	50	20.6 (19.0–22.2)
29	14.5 (13.9–15.2)	51	20.9 (19.3–22.5)
30	14.8 (14.1–15.5)	52	21.2 (19.5–22.9)
31	15.1 (14.3–15.9)	53	21.5 (19.8–23.2)
32	15.3 (14.5–16.1)	54	21.9 (20.1–23.7)
33	15.6 (14.7–16.5)	55	22.2 (20.4–24.0)
34	15.9 (15.0–16.8)	56	22.5 (20.7–24.3)
35	16.2 (15.2–17.2)	57	22.8 (21.1–24.5)
36	16.4 (15.4–17.4)	58	23.2 (21.5–24.9)
37	16.7 (15.6–17.8)	59	23.5 (21.9–25.1)
38	17.0 (15.9–18.1)	60	23.8 (22.3–25.5)
39	17.3 (16.1–18.5)	61	24.2 (22.6–25.8)
40	17.6 (16.4–18.8)	62	24.6 (23.1–26.1)
41	17.9 (16.5–19.3)	63	24.9 (23.4–26.4)

Biparietal diameter (mm)	Gestational age (weeks, mean[a] and range[b])	Biparietal diameter (mm)	Gestational age (weeks, mean[a] and range[b])
64	25.3 (23.8–26.8)	82	32.6 (31.2–34.0)
65	25.6 (24.1–27.1)	83	33.0 (31.5–34.5)
66	26.0 (24.5–27.5)	84	33.4 (31.9–35.1)
67	26.4 (25.0–27.8)	85	34.0 (32.3–35.7)
68	26.7 (25.3–28.1)	86	34.3 (32.8–36.2)
69	27.1 (25.8–28.4)	87	35.0 (33.4–36.6)
70	27.5 (26.3–28.7)	88	35.4 (33.9–37.1)
71	27.9 (26.7–29.1)	89	36.1 (34.6–37.6)
72	28.3 (27.2–29.4)	90	36.6 (35.1–38.1)
73	28.7 (27.6–29.8)	91	37.2 (35.9–38.5)
74	29.1 (28.1–30.1)	92	37.8 (36.7–38.9)
75	29.5 (28.5–30.5)	93	38.8 (37.3–39.3)
76	30.0 (29.0–31.0)	94	39.0 (37.9–40.1)
77	30.3 (29.2–31.4)	95	39.7 (38.5–40.9)
78	30.8 (29.6–32.0)	96	40.6 (39.1–41.5)
79	31.1 (29.9–32.5)	97	41.0 (39.9–42.1)
80	31.6 (30.2–33.0)	98	41.8 (40.5–43.1)
81	32.1 (30.7–33.5)		

[a] Weighted least mean square fit equation: BPD (mm) $-34.5701 + 5.0157GA - 0.0441GA^2$ (where BPD is the biparietal diameter and GA is the mean gestational age).
[b] 90% variation.

FURTHER READING
Kurtz AB, Wapner RJ, Kurtz RJ, Dershaw DD, Rubin CS, Cole-Beuglet C, Goldberg BB. Analysis of biparietal diameter as an accurate indicator of gestational age. *Journal of Clinical Ultrasound* 1980;**8**:319–326.

Head circumference

PREPARATION
Full bladder for transabdominal imaging in first and second trimester.

POSITION
Transaxial image of fetal skull at level of thalami and cavum septum pellucidum, parallel to the skull base.

PROBE
3.0–5.0 MHz transducer is used for all second- and third-trimester obstetric imaging.

METHOD
Outer perimeter of cranium. Alternatively it can be calculated by the following formula:

$$1.57 \times ([\text{outer-to-outer BPD}] + [\text{outer-to-outer OFD}])$$

where BPD is the biparietal diameter and OFD is the occipitofrontal diameter.

APPEARANCE
Thalami appear as symmetric low-reflective structures on either side of linear midline high-reflective line (third ventricle). Calvaria must appear smooth and symmetric bilaterally. The cavum septum pellucidi must be visible anteriorly and the tentorial hiatus posteriorly.

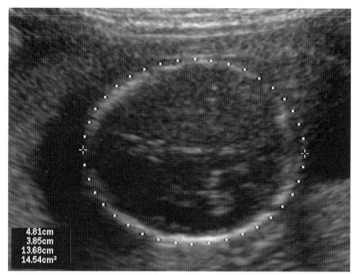

4.81cm
3.85cm
13.68cm
14.54cm²

Figure 99 In the axial plane at the level of the thalami and the cavum septum pellucidum, parallel to the skull base, an outer perimeter of the cranium is constructed

MEASUREMENTS

Head circumference (mm)	Gestational age (weeks, mean and 95%CI)	Head circumference (mm)	Gestational age (weeks, mean and 95%CI)
80	13.4 (12.1–14.7)	190	21.2 (19.8–22.8)
85	13.7 (12.4–15.0)	195	21.6 (20.0–23.2)
90	14.0 (12.7–15.3)	200	22.1 (20.5–23.7)
95	14.3 (13.0–15.6)	205	22.5 (20.9–24.1)
100	14.6 (13.3–15.9)	210	23.0 (21.4–24.6)
105	15.0 (13.7–16.3)	215	23.4 (21.8–25.0)
110	15.3 (14.0–16.6)	220	23.9 (22.3–25.5)
115	15.6 (14.3–16.9)	225	24.4 (22.1–26.7)
120	15.9 (14.6–17.2)	230	24.9 (22.6–27.2)
125	16.3 (15.0–17.6)	235	25.4 (23.1–27.7)
130	16.6 (15.3–17.9)	240	25.9 (23.6–28.2)
135	17.0 (15.7–18.3)	245	26.4 (24.1–28.7)
140	17.3 (16.0–18.6)	250	26.9 (24.6–29.2)
145	17.7 (16.4–19.0)	255	27.5 (25.2–29.8)
150	18.1 (16.5–19.7)	260	28.0 (25.7–30.3)
155	18.4 (16.8–20.0)	265	28.1 (25.8–30.4)
160	18.8 (17.2–20.4)	270	29.2 (26.9–31.5)
165	19.2 (17.6–20.8)	275	29.8 (27.5–32.1)
170	19.6 (18.0–21.2)	280	30.3 (27.6–33.0)
175	20.0 (18.4–21.6)	285	31.0 (28.3–33.7)
180	20.4 (18.8–22.0)	290	31.6 (28.9–34.3)
185	20.8 (19.2–22.4)	295	32.2 (29.5–34.8)

Head circumference (mm)	Gestational age (weeks, mean and 95%CI)	Head circumference (mm)	Gestational age (weeks, mean and 95%CI)
300	32.8 (30.1–35.5)	335	37.7 (34.3–41.1)
305	33.5 (30.7–36.2)	340	38.5 (35.1–41.9)
310	34.2 (31.5–36.9)	345	39.2 (35.8–42.6)
315	34.9 (32.2–37.6)	350	40.0 (36.6–43.4)
320	35.5 (32.8–38.2)	355	40.8 (37.4–44.2)
325	36.3 (32.9–39.7)	360	41.6 (38.2–45.0)
330	37.0 (33.6–40.0)		

FURTHER READING

Hadlock FP, Deter RL, Harrist RB, Park SK. Fetal head circumference: relation to menstrual age. *American Journal of Roentgenology* 1982;**138**:649–653.

Abdominal circumference

PREPARATION
Full bladder for transabdominal imaging in first and second trimester.

POSITION
Transverse image of fetal abdomen at level of the stomach and intra-hepatic umbilical vein.

PROBE
3.0–5.0 MHz transabdominal transducer is used for all second- and third-trimester obstetric imaging.

METHOD
Length of outer perimeter of fetal abdomen.

APPEARANCE
In the correct plane, the abdomen should appear round (rather than elliptical), the ribs are symmetric and the confluence of the right and left portal veins and the fetal stomach should be visible. The intra-hepatic umbilical vein appears in short axis.

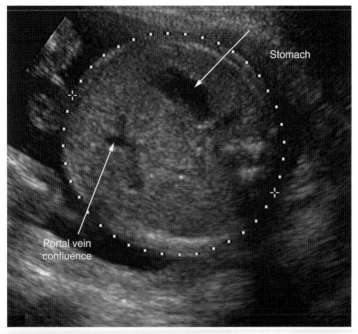

Figure 100 Abdominal circumference is obtained by placing electronic cursors around the perimeter of the fetal abdomen at the level of the stomach, intrahepatic umbilical vein and confluence of the right and left portal veins

MEASUREMENTS

Abdominal circumference (mm)	Gestational age (weeks, mean and 95%CI)	Abdominal circumference (mm)	Gestational age (weeks, mean and 95%CI)
100	15.6 (13.7–17.5)	210	25.4 (23.2–27.6)
105	16.1 (14.2–18.0)	215	25.9 (23.7–28.1)
110	16.5 (14.6–18.4)	220	26.3 (24.1–28.5)
115	16.9 (15.0–18.8)	225	26.8 (24.6–29.0)
120	17.3 (15.4–19.2)	230	27.3 (25.1–29.5)
125	17.8 (15.9–19.7)	235	27.7 (25.5–29.9)
130	18.2 (16.2–20.2)	240	28.2 (26.0–30.4)
135	18.6 (16.6–20.6)	245	28.7 (26.5–30.9)
140	19.1 (17.1–21.1)	250	29.2 (27.0–31.4)
145	19.5 (17.5–21.5)	255	29.7 (27.5–31.9)
150	20.0 (18.0–22.0)	260	30.1 (27.1–33.1)
155	20.4 (18.4–22.4)	265	30.6 (27.6–33.6)
160	20.8 (18.8–22.8)	270	31.1 (28.1–34.1)
165	21.3 (19.3–23.3)	275	31.6 (28.6–34.6)
170	21.7 (19.7–23.7)	280	32.1 (29.1–35.1)
175	22.2 (20.2–24.2)	285	32.6 (29.6–35.6)
180	22.6 (20.6–24.6)	290	33.1 (30.1–36.1)
185	23.1 (21.1–25.1)	295	33.6 (30.6–36.6)
190	23.6 (21.6–25.6)	300	34.1 (31.1–37.1)
195	24.0 (21.8–26.2)	305	34.6 (31.1–37.1)
200	24.5 (22.3–26.7)	310	35.1 (32.1–38.1)
205	24.9 (22.7–27.1)	315	35.6 (32.6–38.6)

Abdominal circumference (mm)	Gestational age (weeks, mean and 95%CI)	Abdominal circumference (mm)	Gestational age (weeks, mean and 95%CI)
320	36.1 (33.6–38.6)	345	38.7 (36.2–41.2)
325	36.6 (34.1–39.1)	350	39.2 (36.7–41.7)
330	37.1 (34.6–39.6)	355	39.7 (37.2–42.2)
335	37.6 (35.1–40.1)	360	40.2 (37.7–42.7)
340	38.1 (35.6–40.6)	365	40.8 (38.3–43.3)

Further reading

From Hadlock FP, Deter RL, Harrist RB, Park SK. Fetal abdominal circumference as a predictor of menstrual age. *American Journal of Roentgenology* 1982;**139**:367–370.

Multiple fetal parameters in the assessment of gestational age

PREPARATION
Full bladder for transabdominal imaging in first and second trimester.

PROBE
3.0–5.0 MHz transabdominal transducer is used for all second- and third-trimester obstetric imaging

METHOD
Take the mean measurements for the four parameters – biparietal diameter, head circumference, abdominal circumference, femur length. Find the mean gestational ages of each, add them together and divide by four.

MEASUREMENTS

Mean gestational age (weeks)	Mean biparietal diameter (mm)	Mean head circumference (mm)	Mean abdominal circumference (mm)	Mean Femur Length (mm)
12.0	17	68	46	7
12.5	19	75	53	9
13.0	21	82	60	11
13.5	23	89	67	12
14.0	25	97	73	14
14.5	27	104	80	16
15.0	29	110	86	17
15.5	31	117	93	19
16.0	32	124	99	20
16.5	34	131	106	22
17.0	36	138	112	24
17.5	38	144	119	25
18.0	39	151	125	27
18.5	41	158	131	28
19.0	43	164	137	30
19.5	45	170	144	31
20.0	46	177	150	33
20.5	48	183	156	34
21.0	50	189	162	35
21.5	51	195	168	37
22.0	53	201	174	38
22.5	55	207	179	40

Mean gestational age (weeks)	Mean biparietal diameter (mm)	Mean head circumference (mm)	Mean abdominal circumference (mm)	Mean Femur Length (mm)
23.0	56	213	185	41
23.5	58	219	191	42
24.0	59	224	197	44
24.5	61	230	202	45
25.0	62	235	208	46
25.5	64	241	213	47
26.0	65	246	219	49
26.5	67	251	224	50
27.0	68	256	230	51
27.5	69	261	235	52
28.0	71	266	240	54
28.5	72	271	246	55
29.0	73	275	251	56
29.5	75	280	256	57
30.0	76	284	261	58
30.5	77	288	266	59
31.0	78	293	271	60
31.5	79	297	276	61
32.0	81	301	281	62
32.5	82	304	286	63
33.0	83	308	291	64
33.5	84	312	295	65
34.0	85	315	300	66

Mean gestational age (weeks)	Mean biparietal diameter (mm)	Mean head circumference (mm)	Mean abdominal circumference (mm)	Mean Femur Length (mm)
34.5	86	318	305	67
35.0	87	322	309	68
35.5	88	325	314	69
36.0	89	328	318	70
36.5	89	330	323	71
37.0	90	333	327	72
37.5	91	335	332	73
38.0	92	338	336	74
38.5	92	340	340	74
39.0	93	342	344	75
39.5	94	344	348	76
40.0	94	346	353	77

FURTHER READING

From Hadlock FP, Deter RL, Harrist RB, Park SK. Estimated fetal age: computer-assisted analysis of multiple fetal growth parameters. *Radiology* 1984;**152**:497–501.

Ratio of head to abdomen circumference

PREPARATION
Full bladder for transabdominal imaging in first and second trimester.

POSITION
Transaxial image of fetal skull at level of thalami and cavum septum pellucidum. Transverse image of fetal abdomen at level of the stomach and intrahepatic umbilical vein.

PROBE
3.0–5.0 MHz transabdominal transducer is used for all second- and third-trimester obstetric imaging.

METHOD
Outer perimeter of cranium. Length of outer perimeter of fetal abdomen. Elevated head to abdomen circumference ratio is a sign of intrauterine growth retardation (small for gestational age).

APPEARANCE
Thalami appear as symmetric low-reflective structures on either side of linear midline high-reflective line (third ventricle). Calvaria must appear smooth and symmetric bilaterally. The cavum septum pellucidi must be visible anteriorly and the tentorial hiatus posteriorly. In the correct plane, the abdomen should appear round (rather than elliptical), the ribs are symmetric and the confluence of the right and left portal veins and the fetal stomach should be visible. The intrahepatic umbilical vein appears in short axis

MEASUREMENTS

Gestational age (weeks)	Head circumference/ abdominal circumference (mean and range from 5th to 95th percentile)
13–14	1.23 (1.14–1.31)
15–16	1.22 (1.05–1.39)
17–18	1.18 (1.07–1.29)
19–20	1.18 (1.09–1.39
21–22	1.15 (1.06–1.25)
23–24	1.13 (1.05–1.21)
25–26	1.13 (1.04–1.22)
27–28	1.13 (1.05–1.21)
29–30	1.10 (0.99–1.21)
31–32	1.07 (0.96–1.17)
33–34	1.04 (0.96–1.1)
35–36	1.02 (0.93–1.11)
37–38	0.98 (0.92–1.05)
39–40	0.97 (0.87–1.06)
41–42	0.96 (0.93–1.00)

FURTHER READING
From Hadlock FP, Deter RL, Harrist RB, Park SK. Fetal abdominal circumference as a predictor of menstrual age. *American Journal of Roentgenology* 1982;**139**:367–370.

Estimated fetal weight based on biparietal diameter and abdominal circumference

PREPARATION
Full bladder for transabdominal imaging in first and second trimester.

PROBE
3.0–5.0 MHz transabdominal transducer is used for all second- and third-trimester obstetric imaging/

METHOD

$$\log (BW) = -1.7492 + 0.166\ BPD + 0.046\ AC) - 0.00264\ (AC \times BPD)$$

where AC is the abdominal circumference, BPD is the biparietal diameter and BW is the birth weight (in grams).

Abdominal circumference (mm)

BPD (mm)	155	160	165	170	175	180	185	190	195	200	205	210	215
31	224	234	244	255	267	279	291	304	318	332	346	362	378
32	231	241	251	263	274	286	299	312	326	340	355	371	388
33	237	248	259	270	282	294	307	321	335	349	365	381	397
34	244	255	266	278	290	302	316	329	344	359	374	391	408
35	251	262	274	285	298	311	324	338	353	368	384	401	418
36	259	270	281	294	306	319	333	347	362	378	394	411	429
37	266	278	290	302	315	328	342	357	372	388	404	422	440
38	274	286	298	310	324	337	352	366	382	398	415	432	451
39	282	294	306	319	333	347	361	376	392	409	426	444	462
40	290	303	315	328	342	356	371	386	403	419	437	455	474
41	299	311	324	338	352	366	381	397	413	430	448	467	486
42	308	320	333	347	361	376	392	408	424	442	460	479	498
43	317	330	343	357	371	387	402	419	436	453	472	491	511
44	326	339	353	367	382	397	413	430	447	465	484	504	524
45	335	349	363	377	393	408	425	442	459	478	497	517	538
46	345	359	373	386	404	420	436	454	472	490	510	530	551
47	355	369	384	399	415	431	448	466	484	503	524	544	565
48	366	380	395	410	426	443	460	478	497	517	537	558	580
49	376	391	406	422	438	455	473	491	510	530	551	572	594
50	387	402	418	434	451	468	486	505	524	544	565	587	610
51	399	414	430	446	463	481	499	518	538	559	580	602	625
52	410	426	442	459	476	494	513	532	552	573	595	618	641
53	422	438	455	472	489	508	527	547	567	589	611	634	657
54	435	451	468	485	503	522	541	561	582	604	627	650	674
55	447	464	481	499	517	536	556	577	598	620	643	667	691
56	461	477	495	513	532	551	571	592	614	636	660	684	709
57	474	491	509	527	547	566	587	608	630	653	677	701	727
58	488	505	524	542	562	582	603	625	647	670	695	719	745
59	502	520	539	558	578	598	619	642	664	688	713	738	764
60	517	535	554	573	594	615	636	659	682	706	731	757	784
61	532	550	570	590	610	632	654	677	700	725	750	777	804
62	547	566	586	606	627	649	672	695	719	744	770	797	824
63	563	583	603	624	645	667	690	714	738	764	790	817	845
64	580	600	620	641	663	686	709	733	758	784	811	838	867
65	597	617	638	659	682	705	728	753	778	805	832	860	889
66	614	635	656	678	701	724	748	773	799	826	853	882	911
67	632	653	675	697	720	744	769	794	820	848	876	905	935
68	651	672	694	717	740	765	790	816	842	870	898	928	958
69	670	691	714	737	761	786	811	838	865	893	922	952	983
70	689	711	734	758	782	807	833	860	888	916	946	976	1008

Abdominal circumference (mm)

BPD (mm)	155	160	165	170	175	180	185	190	195	200	205	210	215
71	709	732	755	779	804	830	856	883	912	941	971	1002	1033
72	730	763	777	801	827	853	880	907	936	965	996	1027	1060
73	751	775	799	824	850	876	904	932	961	991	1022	1054	1087
74	773	797	822	847	874	901	928	957	987	1017	1049	1081	1114
75	796	820	845	871	898	925	954	983	1013	10'	1076	1109	1143
76	819	844	870	896	923	951	980	1009	1040	1072	1104	1137	1172
77	843	868	894	921	949	977	1007	1037	1068	1100	1133	1167	1202
78	868	894	920	947	975	1004	1034	1065	1096	1129	1162	1197	1232
79	893	919	946	974	1003	1032	1062	1094	1126	1159	1193	1228	1264
80	919	946	973	1002	1031	1061	1091	1123	1156	1189	1224	1259	1296
81	946	973	1001	1030	1060	1090	1121	1153	1187	1221	1256	1292	1329
82	974	1001	1030	1059	1089	1120	1152	1185	1218	1253	1288	1325	1363
83	1002	1030	1059	1089	1120	1151	1183	1217	1251	1286	1322	1359	1397
84	1032	1060	1090	1120	1151	1183	1216	1249	1284	1320	1356	1394	1433
85	1062	1091	1121	1151	1183	1216	1249	1283	1318	1355	1392	1430	1469
86	1093	1122	1153	1184	1216	1249	1283	1318	1354	1390	1428	1467	1507
87	1125	1155	1186	1218	1250	1284	1318	1353	1390	1427	1465	1505	1545
88	1157	1188	1220	1252	1285	1319	1354	1390	1427	1465	1504	1543	1584
89	1191	1222	1254	1287	1321	1356	1391	1428	1465	1503	1543	1583	1625
90	1226	1258	1290	1324	1358	1393	1429	1456	1504	1543	1583	1624	1666
91	1262	1294	1327	1361	1396	1432	1468	1506	1544	1584	1624	1666	1708
92	1299	1332	1365	1400	1435	1471	1508	1546	1586	1626	1667	1709	1752
93	1337	1370	1404	1439	1475	1512	1550	1588	1628	1668	1710	1753	1796
94	1376	1410	1444	1480	1516	1554	1592	1631	1671	1712	1755	1798	1842
95	1416	1450	1486	1522	1559	1597	1635	1675	1716	1758	1800	1844	1889
96	1457	1492	1528	1565	1602	1641	1680	1720	1762	1804	1847	1892	1937
97	1500	1535	1572	1609	1547	1686	1726	1767	1809	1852	1895	1940	1986
98	1544	1580	1617	1654	1693	1733	1773	1815	1857	1900	1945	1990	2037
99	1589	1625	1663	1701	1740	1781	1822	1864	1907	1951	1996	2042	2089
100	1635	1672	1710	1749	1789	1830	1871	1914	1958	2002	2048	2094	2142

Abdominal Circumference (mm)

BPD(mm)	220	225	230	235	240	245	250	255	260	265	270	275	280
31	395	412	431	450	470	491	513	536	559	584	610	638	666
32	405	423	441	461	481	502	525	548	572	597	624	651	680
33	415	433	452	472	493	514	537	560	585	611	638	666	693
34	425	444	463	483	504	526	549	573	598	624	652	680	710
35	436	455	475	495	517	539	562	587	612	638	666	695	725
36	447	466	486	507	529	552	575	600	626	653	681	710	740
37	458	478	498	519	542	565	589	614	640	667	696	725	756
38	470	490	510	532	554	578	602	628	654	682	711	741	772
39	482	502	523	545	568	592	616	642	669	697	727	757	789
40	494	514	536	558	581	606	631	657	684	713	743	773	806
41	506	527	549	572	595	620	645	672	700	729	759	790	828
42	519	540	562	585	609	634	660	688	716	745	776	807	841
43	532	554	576	600	624	649	676	703	732	762	793	825	859
44	545	567	590	614	639	665	692	719	749	779	810	843	877
45	559	581	605	629	654	680	708	736	765	796	828	861	896
46	573	596	620	644	670	696	724	753	783	814	846	880	915
47	588	611	635	660	686	713	741	770	801	832	865	899	934
48	602	626	650	676	702	730	758	788	819	851	884	919	954
49	617	641	666	692	719	747	776	806	837	870	903	938	975
50	633	657	683	709	736	765	794	824	856	889	923	959	996
51	649	674	699	726	754	783	$12	843	876	909	944	980	1017
52	665	690	717	744	772	801	831	863	895	929	964	1001	1039
53	682	708	734	762	790	820	851	883	916	950	986	1023	1061
54	699	725	752	780	809	839	870	903	936	971	1007	1045	1084
55	717	743	771	799	828	859	891	924	958	993	1030	1068	1107
56	735	762	789	818	848	879	911	945	979	1015	1052	1091	1131
57	753	780	809	838	869	900	933	966	1001	1038	1075	1114	1155
58	772	800	829	858	889	921	964	989	1024	1061	1099	1139	1180
59	792	820	849	879	911	943	977	1011	1047	1085	1123	1163	1205
60		840	870	900	932	965	999	1035	1071	1109	1148	1189	1231
61	832	861	891	922	955	988	1023	1058	1095	1134	1173	1214	1257
62	853	882	913	945	977	1011	1046	1083	1120	1159	1199	1241	1284
63	874	904	935	967	1001	1035	1071	1107	1145	1185	1226	1268	1311
64	896	927	958	991	1025	1059	1096	1133	1171	1211	1253	1295	1339
65	919	950	982	1015	1049	1084	1121	1159	1198	1238	1280	1323	1368
66	942	973	1006	1039	1074	1110	1147	1185	1225	1266	1308	1352	1397
67	965	997	1030	1065	1100	1136	1174	1213	1253	1294	1337	1381	1427
68	990	1022	1056	1090	1126	1163	1201	1241	1281	1323	1367	1411	1458
69	1015	1048	1082	1117	1153	1190	1229	1269	1310	1353	1397	1442	1489
70	1040	1074	1108	1144	1181	1219	1258	1298	1340	1383	1427	1473	1521

Abdominal Circumference (mm)

BPD(mm)	220	225	230	235	240	245	250	255	260	265	270	275	280
71	1066	1100	1135	1171	1209	1247	1287	1328	1370	1414	1459	1505	1553
72	1093	1128	1163	1200	1238	1277	1317	1358	1401	1445	1491	1538	1586
73	1121	1156	1192	1229	1267	1307	1348	1390	1433	1478	1524	1571	1620
74	1149	1184	1221	1259	1297	1338	1379	1421	1465	1511	1557	1605	1655
75	1178	1214	1251	1289	1328	1369	1411	1454	1499	1544	1592	1640	1690
76	1207	1244	1281	1320	1360	1401	1444	1487	1533	1579	1627	1676	1727
77	1238	1275	1313	1352	1393	1434	1477	1522	1567	1614	1663	1712	1764
78	1269	1306	1345	1385	1426	1468	1512	1557	1603	1650	1699	1749	1801
79	1301	1339	1378	1418	1460	1503	1547	1592	1639	1687	1737	1787	1840
80	1333	1372	1412	1453	1495	1538	1583	1629	1676	1725	1775	1826	1879
81	1367	1406	1446	1488	1531	1575	1620	1666	1714	1763	1814	1866	1919
82	1401	1441	1482	1524	1567	1612	1657	1704	1753	1803	1854	1906	1960
83	1436	1477	1518	1561	1605	1650	1696	1744	1793	1843	1895	1948	2002
84	1473	1513	1555	1599	1643	1689	1735	1784	1833	1884	1936	1990	2045
85	1510	1551	1594	1637	1682	1728	1776	1825	1875	1926	1979	2033	2089
86	1548	1589	1633	1677	1722	1769	1817	1866	1917	1969	2022	2077	2134
87	1586	1629	1673	1717	1764	1811	1859	1909	1960	2013	2067	2122	2179
88	1626	1669	1714	1759	1806	1854	1903	1953	2005	2058	2113	2169	2226
89	1667	1711	1756	1802	1849	1897	1947	1998	2050	2104	2159	2216	2274
90	1709	1753	1799	1845	1893	1942	1992	2044	2097	2151	2207	2264	2322
91	1752	1797	1843	1890	1938	1988	2039	2091	2144	2199	2255	2313	2372
92	1796	1841	1888	1936	1984	2035	2086	2139	2193	2248	2305	2363	2423
93	1841	1887	1934	1982	2032	2083	2135	2188	2242	2298	2356	2414	2475
94	1887	1934	1982	2030	2080	2132	2184	2238	2293	2350	2407	2467	2527
95	1935	1982	2030	2080	2130	2182	2235	2289	2345	2402	2460	2520	2582
96	1984	2031	2080	2130	2181	2233	2287	2342	2398	2456	2515	2575	2637
97	2033	2082	2131	2181	2233	2286	2340	2396	2452	2510	2570	2631	2693
98	2085	2133	2183	2234	2286	2340	2395	2451	2508	2567	2627	2688	2751
99	2137	2186	2237	2288	2341	2395	2450	2507	2565	2624	2684	2746	2810
100	2191	2241	2292	2344	2397	2452	2507	2564	2623	2682	2743	2806	2870

Abdominal Circumference (mm)

BPD (mm)	285	290	295	300	305	310	315	320	325	330	335	340	345
31	696	726	759	793	828	865	903	943	985	1029	1075	1123	1173
32	710	742	774	809	844	882	921	961	1004	1048	1094	1143	1193
33	725	757	790	825	861	899	938	979	1022	1067	1114	1163	1214
34	740	773	806	841	878	916	956	998	1041	1087	1134	1183	1235
35	756	789	823	858	896	934	975	1017	1061	1107	1154	1204	1256
36	772	805	840	876	913	953	993	1036	1080	1127	1175	1226	1278
37	788	822	857	893	931	971	1012	1056	1101	1147	1196	1247	1300
38	805	839	874	911	950	990	1032	1076	1121	1168	1218	1269	1323
39	822	856	892	930	969	1009	1052	1096	1142	1190	1240	1292	1346
40	839	874	911	949	988	1029	1072	1117	1163	1212	1262	1315	1369
41	857	892	929	968	1008	1049	1093	1138	1185	1234	1285	1338	1393
42	875	911	948	987	1028	1070	1114	1159	1207	1256	1308	1361	1417
43	893	930	968	1007	1048	1091	1135	1181	1229	1279	1331	1385	1442
44	912	949	987	1027	1069	1112	1157	1204	1252	1303	1355	1410	1467
45	932	969	1008	1048	1090	1134	1179	1226	1275	1326	1380	1435	1492
46	951	989	1028	1069	1112	1156	1202	1249	1299	1351	1404	1406	1618
47	971	1010	1049	1091	1134	1178	1225	1273	1323	1375	1430	1486	1545
48	992	1031	1071	1113	1156	1201	1248	1297	1348	1401	1455	1512	1571
49	1013	1052	1093	1135	1179	1225	1272	1322	1373	1426	1482	1539	1599
50	1034	1074	1115	1158	1203	1249	1297	1347	1399	1452	1508	1566	1626
51	1056	1096	1138	1181	1226	1273	1322	1372	1425	1479	1535	1594	1655
52	1078	1119	1161	1205	1251	1298	1347	1398	1451	1506	1563	1622	1683
53	1101	1142	1185	1229	1276	1323	1373	1425	1478	1533	1591	1651	1713
54	1124	1166	1209	1254	1301	1349	1399	1452	1506	1562	1620	1680	1742
55	1148	1190	1234	1279	1327	1376	1426	1479	1534	1590	1649	1710	1773
56	1172	1215	1259	1305	1353	1402	1454	1507	1562	1619	1678	1740	1803
57	1197	1240	1285	1332	1380	1430	1482	1535	1591	1649	1709	1770	1835
58	1222	1266	1311	1358	1407	1458	1510	1564	1621	1679	1739	1802	1866
59	1248	1292	1338	1386	1435	1486	1539	1594	1651	1710	1770	1834	1899
60	1274	1319	1366	1414	1464	1515	1569	1624	1682	1741	1802	1866	1932
61	1301	1346	1393	1442	1493	1545	1599	1655	1713	1773	1835	1899	1965
62	1328	1374	1422	1471	1522	1575	1630	1686	1745	1805	1868	1932	1999
63	1356	1403	1451	1501	1552	1606	1661	1718	1777	1838	1901	1967	2034
64	1385	1432	1481	1531	1583	1637	1693	1751	1810	1872	1935	2001	2069
65	1414	1462	1511	1562	1615	1669	1725	1784	1844	1906	1970	2037	2105
66	1444	1492	1542	1594	1647	1702	1759	1817	1878	1941	2006	2073	2142
67	1474	1523	1574	1626	1679	1735	1792	1852	1913	1976	2042	2109	2179
68	1505	1555	1606	1658	1713	1769	1827	1887	1949	2012	2078	2147	2217
69	1537	1587	1639	1692	1747	1803	1862	1922	1985	2049	2116	2184	2255
70	1570	1620	1672	1726	1781	1839	1898	1959	2022	2087	2154	2223	2295

Abdominal Circumference (mm)

BPD (mm)	285	290	295	300	305	310	315	320	325	330	335	340	345
71	1603	1654	1706	1761	1817	1875	1934	1996	2059	2125	2193	2262	2334
72	1636	1688	1741	1796	1853	1911	1971	2044	2098	2164	2232	2302	2375
73	1671	1723	1777	1832	1890	1948	2009	2072	2137	2203	2272	2343	2416
74	1706	1759	1813	1869	1927	1987	2048	2111	2176	2244	2313	2384	2458
75	1742	1795	1850	1907	1965	2025	2087	2151	2217	2265	2354	2426	2501
76	1779	1833	1888	1945	2004	2065	2127	2192	2258	2326	2397	2469	2544
77	1816	1871	1927	1985	2044	2105	2168	2233	2300	2369	2440	2513	2588
78	1855	1910	1966	2025	2085	2146	2210	2275	2343	2412	2484	2557	2633
79	1894	1949	2006	2065	2126	2188	2252	2318	2386	2456	2528	2603	2679
80	1934	1990	2048	2107	2168	2231	2296	2362	2431	2501	2574	2649	2725
81	1975	2031	2089	2149	2211	2275	2340	2407	2476	2547	2620	2695	2773
82	2016	2073	2132	2193	2255	2319	2385	2462	2522	2594	2667	2743	2821
83	2059	2116	2174	2237	2300	2364	2431	2499	2569	2641	2715	2791	2870
84	2102	2160	2220	2282	2345	2410	2477	2546	2617	2689	2764	2841	2920
85	2146	2205	2266	2328	2392	2457	2525	2594	2665	2739	2814	2891	2970
86	2192	2251	2312	2375	2439	2505	2573	2643	2715	2789	2864	2942	3022
87	2238	2298	2359	2423	2488	2554	2623	2693	2765	2840	2916	2994	3074
88	2285	2346	2408	2472	2537	2604	2673	2744	2817	2892	2968	3047	3128
89	2333	2394	2457	2521	2587	2655	2725	2796	2869	29'	3021	3101	3182
90	2382	2444	2507	2572	2639	2707	2777	2849	2923	2998	3076	3155	3237
91	2433	2495	2559	2624	2691	2760	2830	2903	2977	3053	3131	3211	3293
92	2484	2547	2611	2677	2744	2814	2885	2958	3032	3109	3187	3268	3350
93	2536	2599	2664	2731	2799	2869	2940	3014	3089	3166	3245	3326	3409
94	2590	2653	2719	2786	2854	2925	2997	3070	3146	3224	3303	3384	3468
95	2644	2709	2774	2842	2911	2982	3054	3129	3205	3283	3362	3444	3528
96	2700	2765	2831	2899	2969	3040	3113	3188	3264	3343	3423	3505	3589
97	2757	2822	2889	2958	3028	3099	3173	3248	3325	3404	3484	3567	3651
98	2815	2881	2948	3017	3088	3160	3234	3309	3387	3466	3547	3630	3715
99	2874	2941	3009	3078	3149	3222	3296	3372	3450	3529	3611	3694	3779
100	2935	3002	3070	3140	3211	3285	3359	3436	3514	3594	3767	3759	3845

Abdominal Circumference (mm)

BPD (mm)	350	355	360	365	370	375	380	385	390	395	400
31	1225	1279	1336	1396	1458	1523	1591	1661	1735	1812	1893
32	1246	1301	1258	1418	1481	1546	1615	1686	1761	1838	1920
33	1267	1323	1381	1441	1504	1570	1639	1711	1786	1865	1946
34	1289	1345	1403	1464	1528	1595	1664	1737	1812	1891	1973
35	1311	1367	1426	1488	1552	1619	1689	1762	1839	1918	2001
36	1333	1390	1450	1512	1577	1645	1715	1789	1865	1945	2029
37	1356	1413	1474	1536	1602	1670	1741	1815	1893	1973	2057
38	1379	1437	1498	1561	1627	1696	1768	1842	1920	2001	2086
39	1402	1461	1523	1586	1653	1722	1794	1870	1948	2030	2115
40	1426	1486	1548	1612	1679	1749	1822	1898	1977	2059	2145
41	1451	1511	1573	1638	1706	1776	1849	1926	2005	2088	2174
42	1475	1536	1599	1664	1733	1804	1878	1954	2035	2118	2205
43	1500	1562	1625	1691	1760	1832	1906	1984	2064	2148	2236
44	1526	1588	1652	1718	1788	1860	1935	2013	2094	2179	2267
45	1552	1614	1679	1746	1816	1889	1964	2043	2125	2210	2298
46	1579	1641	1706	1774	1845	1918	1994	2073	2156	2241	2330
47	1605	1669	1734	1803	1874	1948	2024	2104	2187	2273	2363
48	1633	1697	1763	1832	1904	1976	2055	2136	2219	2306	2396
49	1661	1725	1792	1861	1934	2009	2086	2167	2251	2339	2429
50	1689	1754	1821	1891	1964	2040	2118	2200	2284	2372	2463
51	1718	1783	1851	1922	1995	2071	2150	2232	2317	2406	2498
52	1747	1813	1882	1953	2027	2103	2183	2266	2351	2440	2532
53	1777	1843	1913	1984	2059	2136	2216	2299	2386	2475	2568
54	1807	1874	1944	2016	2091	2169	2250	2333	2420	2510	2604
55	1838	1906	1976	2049	2124	2203	2284	2368	2456	2546	2640
56	1869	1938	2008	2082	2158	2237	2319	2403	2491	2582	2677
57	1901	1970	2041	2115	2192	2272	2354	2439	2528	2619	2714
58	1934	2003	2075	2150	2227	2307	2390	2475	2664	2657	2752
59	1966	2037	2109	2184	2262	2342	2426	2512	2602	2694	2790
60	2000	2071	2144	2219	2298	2379	2463	2550	2640	2733	2829
61	2034	2105	2179	2255	2334	2416	2500	2588	2678	2772	2869
62	2069	2140	2215	2291	2371	2453	2538	2626	2717	2811	2909
63	2104	2176	2251	2328	2408	2491	2577	2665	2757	2851	2949
64	2140	2213	2288	2366	2446	2530	2616	2705	2797	2892	2991
65	2176	2250	2326	2404	2485	2569	2656	2745	2838	2933	3032
66	2213	2287	2364	2443	2524	2609	2696	2786	2879	2975	3075
67	2251	2326	2403	2482	2564	2649	2737	2827	2921	3018	3117
68	2290	2365	2442	2522	2605	2690	2778	2869	2964	3061	3161
69	2329	2404	2482	2563	2646	2732	2821	2912	3007	3104	3205
70	2368	2444	2523	2604	2688	2774	2863	2955	3050	3149	3250

Abdominal Circumference (mm)

BPD (mm)	350	355	360	365	370	375	380	385	390	395	400
71	2409	2485	2564	2646	2730	2817	2907	2999	3095	3193	3295
72	2450	2527	2607	2689	2773	2861	2951	3044	3140	3239	3341
73	2491	2569	2649	2732	2817	2905	2996	3089	3186	3285	3386
74	2534	2612	2693	2776	2862	2950	3041	3135	3232	3332	3435
75	2577	2656	2737	2821	2907	2996	3088	3182	3279	3380	3483
76	2621	2700	2782	2866	2953	3042	3134	3229	3327	3428	3531
77	2666	2746	2828	2912	3000	3090	3128	3277	3376	3477	3581
78	2711	2792	2874	2959	3047	3137	3230	3326	3425	3526	3631
79	2757	2838	2921	3007	3095	3186	3279	3376	3475	3576	3681
80	2804	2886	2969	3056	3144	3235	3329	3426	3525	3627	3733
81	2852	2934	3018	3105	3194	3286	3380	3477	3577	3679	3785
82	2901	2983	3068	3155	3244	3336	3431	3529	3629	3732	3838
83	2950	3033	3118	3206	3296	3388	3483	3581	3682	3785	3891
84	3001	3084	3169	3257	3348	3441	3536	3634	3735	3839	3945
85	3052	3135	3221	3310	3401	3494	3590	3688	3790	3894	4000
86	3104	3188	3274	3363	3454	3548	3644	3743	3845	3949	4056
87	3157	3241	3328	3417	3509	3603	3700	3799	3901	4005	4113
88	3210	3295	3383	3472	3565	3659	3756	3855	3958	4063	4170
89	3265	3351	3438	3528	3621	3716	3813	3913	4015	4120	4228
90	3321	3407	3495	3585	3678	3773	3871	3971	4074	4179	4287
91	3377	3464	3552	3643	3736	3832	3930	4030	4133	4239	4347
92	3435	3522	3611	3702	3795	3891	3989	4090	4193	4299	4408
93	3494	3581	3670	3761	3855	3951	4050	4151	4254	4361	4469
94	3553	3641	3738	3822	3916	4013	4111	4213	4316	4423	4532
95	3614	3701	3791	3884	3978	4075	4174	4275	4379	4486	4595
96	3675	3763	3854	3946	4041	4138	4237	4339	4443	4550	4659
97	3738	3826	3917	4010	4105	4202	4302	4404	4508	4615	4724
98	3802	3890	3981	4074	4170	4267	4367	4469	4573	4680	4790
99	3866	3956	4047	4140	4236	4333	4433	4536	4640	4747	4857
100	3932	4022	4113	4207	4303	4400	4501	4603	4708	4815	4924

FURTHER READING

From Shepard MJ, Richards VA, Berkowitz RL, Warsof SL, Hobbins JC. An evaluation of two equations for predicting fetal weight by ultrasound. *American Journal of Obstetrics and Gynecology* 1982;**147**:47–54.

Fetal femur length

PREPARATION
Full bladder for transabdominal imaging in first and second trimester.

POSITION
Long axis image of fetal femur.

PROBE
3.0–5.0 MHz transabdominal transducer is used for all second- and third-trimester obstetric imaging.

METHOD
Length of ossified diaphysis of femur. Cursor placed at junction of bone and cartilage. Epiphysis should not be measured.

APPEARANCE
The correct position of the transducer along the femoral long axis is confirmed by identifying the femoral condylar epiphysis plus **either** the femoral head epiphysis or greater trochanter within the section plane.

MEASUREMENTS

Femur length (mm)	Gestational age (weeks) Mean and range (5th–95th percentile)
10	12.6 (10.4–14.9)
11	12.9 (10.7–15.1)
12	13.3 (11.1–15.6)
13	13.6 (11.4–15.9)
14	13.9 (11.7–16.1)
15	14.1 (12.0–16.4)
16	14.6 (12.4–16.9)
17	14.9 (12.7–17.1)
18	15.1 (13.0–17.4)
19	15.6 (13.4–17.9)

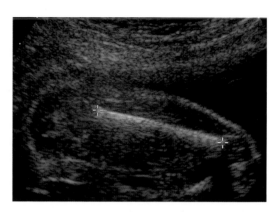

Figure 101 Femur length is obtained by imaging the femur in long axis then placing cursors on each side of the ossified diaphysis of the femur. The epiphysis should not be included

Femur length (mm)	Gestational age (weeks) Mean and range (5th–95th percentile)
20	15.9 (13.7–18.1)
21	16.3 (14.1–18.6)
22	16.6 (14.4–18.9)
23	16.9 (14.7–19.1)
24	17.3 (15.1–19.6)
25	17.6 (15.4–19.9)
26	18.0 (15.9–20.1)
27	18.3 (16.1–20.6)
28	18.7 (16.6–20.9)
29	19.0 (16.9–21.1)
30	19.4 (17.1–21.6)
31	19.9 (17.6–22.0)
32	20.1 (17.9–22.3)
33	20.6 (18.3–22.7)
34	20.9 (18.7–23.1)

Femur length (mm)	Gestational age (weeks) Mean and range (5th–95th percentile)
35	21.1 (19.0–23.4)
36	21.6 (19.4–23.9)
37	22.0 (19.9–24.1)
38	22.4 (20.1–24.6)
39	22.7 (20.6–24.9)
40	23.1 (20.9–25.3)
41	23.6 (21.3–25.7)
42	23.9 (21.7–26.1)
43	24.3 (22.1–26.6)
44	24.7 (22.6–26.9)
45	25.0 (22.9–27.1)
46	25.4 (23.1–27.6)
47	25.9 (23.6–28.0)
48	26.1 (24.0–28.4)
49	26.6 (24.4–28.9)
50	27.0 (24.9–29.1)
51	27.4 (25.1–29.6)
52	27.9 (25.6–30.0)
53	28.1 (26.0–30.4)
54	28.6 (26.4–30.9)
55	29.1 (26.9–31.3)
56	29.6 (27.2–31.7)
57	29.9 (27.7–32.1)
58	30.3 (28.1–32.6)

Femur length (mm)	Gestational age (weeks) Mean and range (5th–95th percentile)
59	30.7 (28.6–32.9)
60	31.1 (28.9–33.3)
61	31.6 (29.4–33.9)
62	32.0 (29.9–34.1)
63	32.4 (30.1–34.6)
64	32.9 (30.7–35.1)
65	33.4 (31.1–35.6)
66	33.7 (31.6–35.9)
67	34.1 (32.0–36.4)
68	34.6 (32.4–36.9)
69	35.0 (32.6–37.1)
70	35.6 (33.3–37.7)
71	35.9 (33.7–38.1)
72	36.4 (34.1–38.6)
73	36.9 (34.6–39.0)
74	37.3 (35.1–39.6)
75	37.7 (35.6–39.9)
76	38.1 (36.0–40.4)
77	38.6 (36.4–40.9)
78	39.1 (36.9–41.3)
79	39.6 (37.3–41.7)

FURTHER READING

Jeanty P, Rodesch F, Delbeke D, Dumont JE. Estimation of gestational age from measurements of fetal long bones. *Journal of Ultrasound in Medicine* 1984;**3**:75–79.

Fetal humerus length

PREPARATION
Full bladder for transabdominal imaging in first and second trimester.

POSITION
Long axis image of fetal humerus.

PROBE
3.0–5.0 MHz transabdominal transducer is used for all second- and third-trimester obstetric imaging.

METHOD
Length of ossified diaphysis of humerus. Cursor placed at junction of bone and cartilage. Epiphysis should not be measured.

APPEARANCE
The correct position of the transducer along the humeral long axis is confirmed by identifying both the proximal and distal epiphyses within the section plane.

Humerus length (mm)	Gestational age (weeks) Mean and range (5th–95th percentile)
10	12.6 (9.9–15.3)
11	12.9 (10.1–15.6)
12	13.1 (10.4–15.9)
13	13.6 (10.9–16.1)
14	13.9 (11.1–16.6)
15	14.1 (11.4–16.9)
16	14.6 (11.9–17.3)
17	14.9 (12.1–17.6)
18	15.1 (12.6–18.0)
19	15.6 (12.9–18.3)

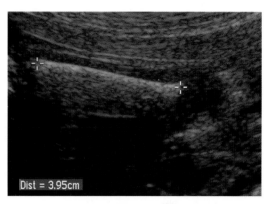

Figure 102 Length of the ossified diaphysis of the humerus, with cursors placed at the junction of bone in cartilage. The epiphysis should not be included (Courtesy of Jane L. Clarke)

Humerus length (mm)	Gestational age (weeks) Mean and range (5th–95th percentile)
20	15.9 (13.1–18.7)
21	16.3 (13.6–19.1)
22	16.7 (13.9–19.4)
23	17.1 (14.3–19.9)
24	17.4 (14.7–20.1)
25	17.9 (15.1–20.6)
26	18.1 (15.6–21.0)
27	18.6 (15.9–21.4)
28	19.0 (16.3–21.9)
29	19.4 (16.7–22.1)
30	19.9 (17.1–22.6)
31	20.3 (17.6–23.0)
32	20.7 (18.0–23.6)
33	21.1 (18.4–23.9)

Humerus length (mm)	Gestational age (weeks) Mean and range (5th–95th percentile)
34	21.6 (18.9–24.3)
35	22.0 (19.3–24.9)
36	22.6 (19.7–25.1)
37	22.9 (20.1–25.7)
38	23.4 (20.6–26.1)
39	23.9 (21.1–26.6)
40	24.3 (21.6–27.1)
41	24.9 (22.0–27.6)
42	25.3 (22.6–28.0)
43	25.7 (23.0–28.6)
44	26.1 (23.6–29.0)
45	26.7 (24.0–29.6)
46	27.1 (24.6–30.0)
47	27.7 (25.0–30.6)
48	28.1 (25.6–31.0)
49	28.9 (26.0–31.6)
50	29.3 (26.6–32.0)
51	29.9 (27.1–32.6)
52	30.3 (27.6–33.1)
53	30.9 (28.1–33.6)
54	31.4 (28.7–34.1)
55	32.0 (29.1–34.7)
56	32.6 (29.9–35.3)

Humerus length (mm)	Gestational age (weeks) Mean and range (5th–95th percentile)
57	33.1 (30.3–35.9)
58	33.6 (30.9–36.4)
59	34.1 (31.4–36.9)
60	34.9 (32.0–37.6)
61	35.3 (32.6–38.1)
62	35.9 (33.1–38.7)
63	36.6 (33.9–39.3)
64	37.1 (34.4–39.9)
65	37.7 (35.0–40.6)
66	38.3 (35.6–41.1)
67	38.9 (36.1–41.7)
68	39.6 (36.9–42.3)
69	40.1 (37.4–42.9)

FURTHER READING

Jeanty P, Rodesch F, Delbeke D, Dumont JE. Estimation of gestational age from measurements of fetal long bones. *Journal of Ultrasound in Medicine* 1984;3:75–79.

Systolic/diastolic ratio in the umbilical artery

PREPARATION
Full bladder for transabdominal imaging in first and second trimester.

POSITION
Spectral Doppler cursor placed on umbilical artery outside the fetus.

PROBE
3.0–5.0 MHz transabdominal transducer is used for all second- and third-trimester obstetric imaging.

METHOD
Spectral Doppler ultrasound recording of umbilical artery peak systolic velocity divided by end diastolic velocity (S/D ratio).

APPEARANCE
Normal umbilical cord contains two arteries and one vein. The vein is larger than the arteries. A single umbilical artery is associated with fetal anomalies.

MEASUREMENTS
Elevated S/D ratios are a sign of placental dysfunction and are associated with intrauterine growth restriction and pregnancy-induced hypertension.

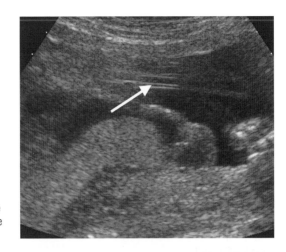

Figure 103a The arrow points to the umbilical vessels

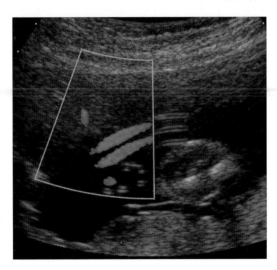

Figure 103b The color Doppler image demonstrates flow in the two umbilical arteries

Gestational age (weeks)	S/D ratio percentiles		
	10%	50%	90%
16	3.01	4.25	6.07
20	3.16	4.04	5.24
24	2.7	3.5	4.75
28	2.41	3.02	3.97
30	2.43	3.04	3.8
32	2.27	2.73	3.57
34	2.08	2.52	3.41
36	1.96	2.35	3.15
38	1.89	2.24	3.1
40	1.83	2.22	2.68
41	1.93	2.21	2.55
42	1.91	2.51	3.21

FURTHER READING

Fogarty P, Beattie B, Harper A, Dornan J. Continuous wave Doppler flow velocity waveforms from the umbilical artery in normal pregnancy. *Journal of Perinatal Medicine* 1990;**18**:51–57.

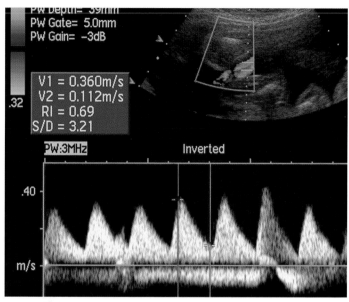

Figure 103c A spectral Doppler gate placed on an umbilical artery returns a normal spectral Doppler waveform, from which the systolic diastolic ratio is calculated (Courtesy of Jane L. Clarke)

Cerebral ventricles – lateral ventricle transverse atrial measurement

PREPARATION
Full bladder for transabdominal imaging in first and second trimester.

POSITION
Axial image obtained at the level of the thalamic nuclei.

PROBE
3.0–5.0 MHz transabdominal transducer is used for all second- and third-trimester obstetric imaging.

METHOD
Transverse atrial measurement taken at confluence of body, occipital and temporal horns of the lateral ventricles. Calipers positioned at level of glomus of the choroid plexus, inside the reflectivity generated by the ventricular walls

APPEARANCE
The choroid plexi is are high-reflective structures filling the atria of the lateral ventricles.

MEASUREMENTS
- The normal value is 7.6 mm between 14 and 38 weeks. Choroid plexi should complete fill the atria.
- Atrial measurement of >10 mm is abnormal and suggestive of hydrocephalus. Choroid plexus that falls away (drooping) from atrial wall is also abnormal even if atrial measurement is <10 mm.

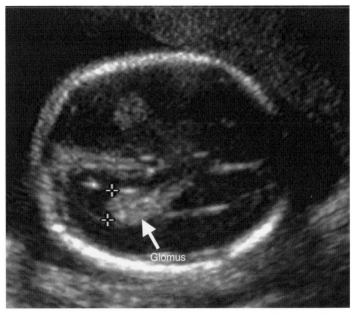

Figure 104 Transverse atrial measurement taken at confluence of body, occipital and temporal horns of the lateral ventricles. Calipers positioned at level of glomus of the choroid plexus, inside the reflectivity generated by the ventricular walls

FURTHER READING

Cardoza JD, Goldstein RB, Filly RA. Exclusion of fetal ventriculomegaly with a single measurement: the width of the lateral ventricular atrium. *Radiology* 1988;**169**:711–714.

15–25 gestational weeks

Pretorius DH, Drose JA, Manco-Johnson ML. Fetal lateral ventricular ratio determined during the second trimester. *Journal of Ultrasound in Medicine* 1986;**5**:121–124.

26 gestational weeks to term

Almog B, Gamzu R, Achiron R, Fainaru O, Zalel Y. Fetal lateral ventricular width: what should be its upper limit? A prospective cohort study and reanalysis of the current and previous data. *Journal of Ultrasound in Medicine* 2003;**22**:39–43.

Johnson ML, Dunne MG, Mack LA, Rashbaum CL. Evaluation of fetal intracranial anatomy by static and real-time ultrasound. *Journal of Ultrasound in Medicine* 1980;**8**:311–318.

Cisterna magna

PREPARATION
Full bladder for transabdominal imaging second trimester.

POSITION
Cerebellar view: transverse axial image with posterior caudal angulation passing through the posterior fossa at level of cerebellum.

PROBE
3.0–5.0 MHz transducer is used for all second- and third-trimester obstetric imaging.

METHOD
Maximum width of the cerebrospinal fluid space between cerebellum and occiput.

APPEARANCE
Fluid-filled space between cerebellum and occiput.

MEASUREMENTS
- Anteroposterior depth (mm) at 15–36 weeks:

Mean	5
Range	2–8
Maximum	10

- Absence of the cisterna magna is suggestive of Chiari malformation.
- Mega-cisterna magna (>10 mm) is associated with chromsomal abnormalities, but can be normal.

FURTHER READING
Mahony BS, Callen PW, Filly RA, Hoddick WK. The fetal cisterna magna. *Radiology* 1984;**153**:773–776.

Figure 105 The cisterna magna measurement is the maximum width of the CSF space between cerebellum and occiput (cursors ×–×). The transverse cerebellar measurement (+–+) and nuchal fold measurement (°– °) are also displayed

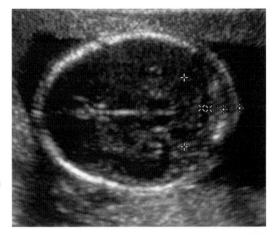

Thoracic circumference

PREPARATION
Full bladder for transabdominal imaging in first and second trimester.

POSITION
Axial image of thorax at the level of the four-chamber heart.

PROBE
3.0–5.0 MHz transducer is used for all second- and third-trimester obstetric imaging.

METHOD
The thoracic circumference, excluding the skin and subcutaneous tissues at the level of the four-chamber view of the heart.

APPEARANCE
Transaxial view through the thorax showing four cardiac chambers.

MEASUREMENTS
- Normal thoracic to abdominal circumference (TC/AC) ratio is 0.89–1.0.
- TC/AC ratio of < 0.8 is associated with pulmonary hypoplasia.

FURTHER READING
Johnson A, Callan NA, Bhutani VK, Colmorgen GH, Weiner S, Bolognese RJ. Ultrasonic ratio of fetal thoracic to abdominal circumference: an association with fetal pulmonary hypoplasia. *American Journal of Obstetrics and Gynecology* 1987;**157**:764–769.

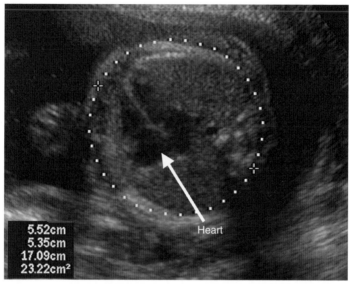

5.52cm
5.35cm
17.09cm
23.22cm²

Heart

Figure 106 An axial image at the level of the four chambers of the heart through the thorax, with a thoracic circumference calculated excluding the skin and subcutaneous tissues

Renal pelvis diameter

PREPARATION
Full bladder for transabdominal imaging in first and second trimester.

POSITION
Transverse image of fetal abdomen at midrenal level.

PROBE
3.0–5.0 MHz transducer is used for all second- and third-trimester obstetric imaging.

METHOD
Anteroposterior diameter measurement of renal pelvis.

APPEARANCE
Fluid filled structure in the centre of the renal sinus. Mild distension of the renal pelvis is normal.

MEASUREMENTS
- *Up to 20 weeks gestation:* <4 mm. ≥4 mm may indicate fetal hydronephrosis and requires follow-up scan in third trimester.
- *After 20 weeks gestation:* 5–9 mm is indeterminate.
- *In third trimester:* 7–9 mm is indeterminate and requires neonatal follow-up.
- Obstruction is more likely if calyceal or ureteral dilatation is also present.
- >10 mm is abnormal

FURTHER READING
Grignon A, Filion R, Filiatrault D, Robitaille P, Homsy Y, Boutin H, Leblond R. Urinary tract dilatation in utero: classification and clinical application. *Radiology* 1986;**160**:645–647.

Mandell J, Blyth RR, Peters CA, Retik AB, Estroff JA, Benacerraf BR. Structural genitourinary defects detected in utero. *Radiology* 1991;178:193.

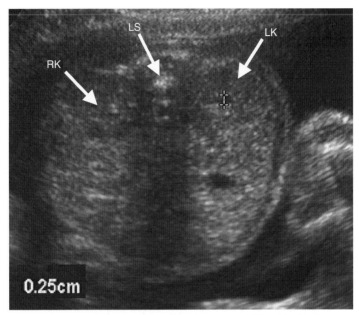

Figure 107 Transverse image of the fetal abdomen at the midrenal level, with an anteroposterior diameter measurement of the renal pelvis. LK, left kidney; LS, lumbar spine; RK, right kidney

Mean renal lengths for gestational ages

PREPARATION
Full bladder for transabdominal imaging in first and second trimester.

POSITION
Sagittal or coronal images of both kidneys.

PROBE
3.0–5.0 MHz transducer is used for all second- and third-trimester obstetric imaging.

METHOD
Maximum long axis measurements. Enlarged kidneys are associated with obstruction, multicystic kidney and polycystic kidney.

APPEARANCE
Elliptical structures with high-reflective margins caused by perirenal fat. Mild pelviectasis is normal.

MEASUREMENTS[1]

Gestational age (weeks)	Length (mm) Mean and 95%CI
18	22 (16–28)
19	23 (15–31)
20	26 (18–34)
21	27 (21–32)
22	27 (20–34)
23	30 (22–37)
24	31 (19–44)
25	33 (25–42)
26	34 (24–44)
27	35 (27–44)
28	34 (26–42)
29	36 (23–48)
30	38 (29–46)

Gestational age (weeks)	Length (mm) Mean and 95%CI
31	37 (28–46)
32	41 (31–51)
33	40 (31–47)
34	42 (33–50)
35	42 (32–52)
36	42 (33–50)
37	42(33–51)
38	44 (32–56)
39	42 (35–48)
40	43 (32–53)
41	45 (39–51)

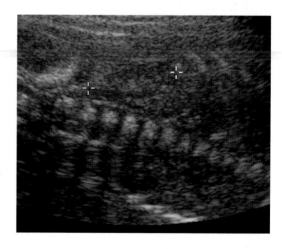

Figure 108
Sagittal image through the kidney (cursors +−+) with the maximum long axis measured (Courtesy of Dr. Maria E.K. Sellars)

REFERENCE
1. Cohen HL, Cooper J, Eisenberg P, Mandel FS, Gross BR, Goldman MA, Barzel E, Rawlinson KF. Normal length of fetal kidneys: Sonographic study in 397 obstetric patients. *American Journal of Roentgenology* 1991;**157**:545–548.

Outer orbital diameter

PREPARATION
Full bladder for transabdominal imaging in first and second trimester.

POSITION
Coronal plane through skull, approximately 2 cm posterior to the glabellar-alveolar line or transverse plane along orbitomeatal line (2–3 cm below biparietal diameter, BPD).

PROBE
3.0–5.0 MHz transducer is used for all second- and third-trimester obstetric imaging.

METHOD
From lateral border of the orbit to opposite lateral border. Can be used in place of BPD when this cannot be measured.

APPEARANCE
The orbits should be symmetric, with both appearing equal and largest possible diameter visualized.

MEASUREMENTS

Binocular distance measurement[1] Predicted outer orbital diameter (mm)	BPD (mm)	Mean gestational age (weeks)
13	19	11.6
14	20	11.6
15	21	12.1
16	22	12.6
17	23	12.6
17	24	13.1
18	25	13.6
19	26	13.6
20	27	14.1
21	28	14.6
21	29	14.6

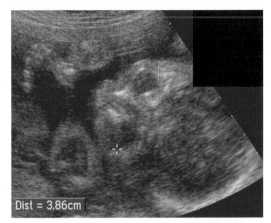

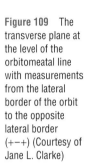

Figure 109 The transverse plane at the level of the orbitomeatal line with measurements from the lateral border of the orbit to the opposite lateral border (+−+) (Courtesy of Jane L. Clarke)

Binocular distance measurement[1] Predicted outer orbital diameter (mm)	BPD (mm)	Mean gestational age (weeks)
22	30	15.0
23	31	15.5
24	32	15.5
25	33	16.0
25	34	16.5
26	35	16.5
27	36	17.0
27	37	17.5
28	38	17.9
30	40	18.4
31	42	18.9
32	43	19.4
32	44	19.4
33	45	19.9
34	46	20.4

Binocular distance measurement[1] Predicted outer orbital diameter (mm)	BPD (mm)	Mean gestational age (weeks)
34	47	20.4
35	48	20.9
36	49	21.3
36	50	21.3
37	51	21.8
38	52	22.3
38	53	22.3
39	54	22.8
40	55	23.3
40	56	23.3
41	57	23.8
41	58	24.3
42	29	24.3
43	60	24.7
43	61	25.2
44	62	25.2
44	63	25.7
45	64	26.2
45	65	26.2
46	66	26.7
46	67	27.2
47	68	27.6
47	69	28.1
48	70	28.6
48	71	29.1
49	73	29.6
50	74	30.0

Binocular distance measurement[1] Predicted outer orbital diameter (mm)	BPD (mm)	Mean gestational age (weeks)
50	75	30.6
51	76	31.0
51	77	31.5
52	78	32.0
52	79	32.5
53	80	33.0
54	82	33.5
54	83	34.5
54	84	34.4
55	85	35.0
55	86	35.4
56	88	35.9
56	89	36.4
57	90	36.9
57	91	37.3
58	92	37.8
58	93	38.3
58	94	38.3
59	96	39.3
59	97	39.8

REFERENCE

1. Mayden KL, Tortora M, Berkowitz RL, Bracken M, Hobbins JC. Orbital diameters: a new parameter for prenatal diagnosis and dating. *American Journal of Obstetrics and Gynecology* 1982;**144**:289–297.

Fetal stomach diameter

PREPARATION
Full bladder for transabdominal imaging in first and second trimester.

POSITION
Long axis, transverse and sagittal images through the fetal stomach.

PROBE
3.0–5.0 MHz transabdominal transducer is used for all second- and third-trimester obstetric imaging.

METHOD
Maximum long axis, transverse and anteroposterior diameters. Enlarged stomach is associated with duodenal atresia.

APPEARANCE
Normal fetal stomach appears as a low-reflective structure on the left side of the abdomen. It should be seen by 13 weeks gestation.

MEASUREMENTS

Gestational age (weeks)	Stomach measurements with range of 5th to 95th percentile[1] (mean ± 2SD, mm)		
	Anteroposterior	Transverse	Longitudinal
13–15	4 (3–5)	6 (4–8)	9 (6–12)
16–18	6 (4–8)	8 (6–10)	13 (9–17)
19–21	8 (6–10)	9 (7–11)	16 (11–21)
22–24	9 (6–12)	18 (15–21)	19 (13–25)
25–27	10 (5–15)	19 (14–24)	23 (13–33)
28–30	12 (9–15)	16 (12–20)	28 (19–37)
31–33	14 (11–17)	16 (12–20)	28 (19–37)
34–36	14 (10–18)	16 (12–20)	28 (19–37)
37–39	16 (12–20)	20 (16–24)	32 (23–41)

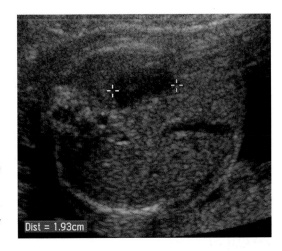

Figure 110
Longitudinal image through the fetal stomach (+−+) measuring the diameter (Courtesy of Jane L. Clarke)

Dist = 1.93cm

REFERENCE

1. Goldstein I, Reece EA, Yarkoni S, Wan M, Green JL, Hobbins JC. Growth of the fetal stomach in normal pregnancies. *Obstetrics and Gynecology* 1987;70:641–644.

Fetal small bowel

PREPARATION
Full bladder for transabdominal imaging in first and second trimester.

POSITION
Short axis image of fluid-filled small bowel.

PROBE
3.0–5.0 MHz transducer is used for all second- and third-trimester obstetric imaging.

METHOD
Maximum diameter of transverse small bowel. Dilated small bowel is associated with volvulus, meconium ileus and jejunal, ileal or colonic atresia.

APPEARANCE
Fluid containing lumen of small bowel is normally seen after 20 weeks.

MEASUREMENTS

Gestational age (weeks)	Transverse diameter of fetal small bowel (mm)[1]	
	Predicted mean value	90th percentile
20–25	1.4	2
25–30	1.8	3
30–35	2.9	6
35–40	3.7	8

FURTHER READING
Parulekar SG. Sonography of normal fetal bowel. *Journal of Ultrasound in Medicine* 1991;**10**:211–220.

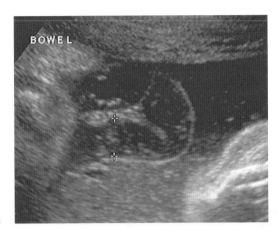

Figure 111 The maximum diameter of transverse small bowel is measured. Fluid-containing lumen of small bowel is normally seen after 20 weeks

REFERENCE
1. Goldstein I, Lockwood C, Hobbins JC. Ultrasound assessment of fetal intestinal development in the evaluation of gestational age. *Obstetrics and Gynecology* 1987;**70**:682–686.

Fetal colon

PREPARATION
Full bladder for transabdominal imaging in first and second trimester.

POSITION
Sagittal view through transverse colon.

PROBE
3.0–5.0 MHz transducer is used for all second- and third-trimester obstetric imaging.

METHOD
For maximum diameter of transverse colon, the colon is measured from outer-to-outer margin. Dilated colon is associated with Hirschsprung's disease, volvulus and colonic atresia.

APPEARANCE
The lumen of normal colon is reliably visualized after 25 weeks.

MEASUREMENTS

Gestational age (weeks)	Transverse diameter of fetal colon (mm)[1]	
	Predicted mean value	90th percentile
26	5	9
30	8	11
35	11	15
40	16	20

REFERENCE
1. Goldstein I, Lockwood C, Hobbins JC: *Ultrasound* assessment of fetal intestinal development in the evaluation of gestational age. *Obstetrics and Gynecology* 1987;70:682–686.

FURTHER READING
Parulekar SG. Sonography of normal fetal bowel. *Journal of Ultrasound in Medicine* 1991;10:211–220.

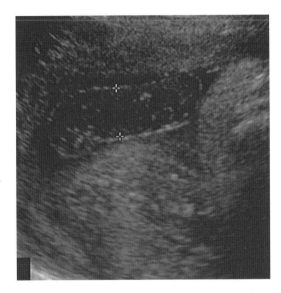

Figure 112 The maximum diameter of transverse colon is measured from outer-to-outer margin. The lumen of normal colon is reliably visualized after 25 weeks

Predicted fetal weight percentiles throughout pregnancy

PREPARATION
Full bladder for transabdominal imaging in first and second trimester.

PROBE
3.0–5.0 MHz transabdominal transducer is used for all second- and third-trimester obstetric imaging.

METHOD

log (BW) = −1.7492 + 0.166 BPD + 0.046 AC) − 0.00264 (AC × BPD)

where AC is the abdominal circumference, BPD is the biparietal diameter and BW is the birth weight (in grams). (Predicted from aborted fetuses 8–21 weeks and births 21–44 weeks.)

MEASUREMENTS

Menstrual weeks	Predicted fetal weight (g), percentiles[1]				
	10	25	50	75	95
8			6.1		
9			7.3		
10			8.1		
11			11.9		
12		11.1	21.1	34.1	
13		22.5	35.3	55.4	
14		34.5	51.4	76.8	
15		51.0	76.7	108	
16		79.8	117	151	
17		125	166	212	
18	280	172	220	298	860
19	320	217	283	394	920
20	370	255	325	460	990
21	420	330	410	570	1080

Menstrual weeks	Predicted fetal weight (g), percentiles[1]				
	10	25	50	75	95
22	490	410	480	630	1180
23	570	460	550	690	1320
24	660	530	640	780	1470
25	770	630	740	890	1660
26	890	730	860	1020	1890
27	1030	840	990	1160	2100
28	1180	980	1150	1350	2290
29	1310	1100	1310	1530	2500
30	1480	1260	1460	1710	2690
31	1670	1410	1630	1880	2880
32	1870	1570	1810	2090	3090
33	2190	1720	2010	2280	3290
34	2310	1910	2220	2510	3470
35	2510	2130	2430	2730	3610
36	2680	2470	2650	2950	3750
37	2750	2580	2870	3160	3870
38	2800	2770	3030	3320	3980
39	2830	2910	3170	3470	4060
40	2840	3010	3280	3590	4100
41	2790	3070	3360	3680	4110
42		3110	3410	3740	
43		3110	3420	3780	
44		3050	3390	3770	

REFERENCE
1. Brenner WE, Edelman DA, Hendricks CH. A standard of fetal growth for the United States of America. *American Journal of Obstetrics and Gynecology* 1976;**126**:555–564.

Amniotic fluid

PREPARATION
None.

POSITION
Uterus is divided into four quadrants using the maternal sagittal mid-line vertically, and an arbitrary transverse line halfway between uterine fundus and upper edge of uterine fundus horizontally.

PROBE
3.0–5.0 MHz transducer is used for all second- and third-trimester obstetric imaging.

METHOD
Transducer is parallel to maternal sagittal plane, and perpendicular to maternal coronal plane. Amniotic fluid index (AFI) is the sum of the maximum vertical depths of the amniotic fluid pockets in the four quadrants. It can be used to determine the volume of amniotic fluid after 16 weeks.

APPEARANCE
The deepest pocket of amniotic fluid in each quadrant is visualized. The pocket should be free of umbilical cord or fetal extremities.

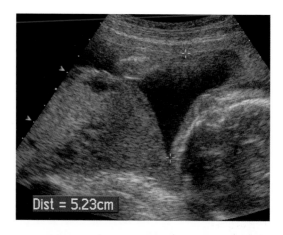

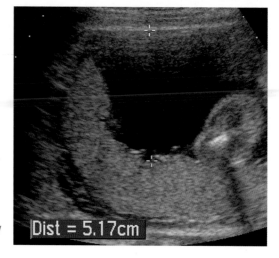

Figure 113 In the sagittal plane measurements are made perpendicular to the maternal coronal plane. Measurements are taken in four quadrants (Courtesy of Jane L. Clarke)

MEASUREMENTS

Gestational age (weeks)	AFI percentile values in normal pregnancy (cm)[1]		
	5th	50th	95th
16	7.9	12.1	18.5
17	8.3	12.7	19.4
18	8.7	13.3	20.2
19	9.0	13.7	20.7
20	9.3	14.1	21.2
21	9.5	14.3	21.4
22	9.7	14.5	21.6
23	9.8	14.6	21.8
24	9.8	14.7	21.9
36	7.7	13.8	24.9
37	7.5	13.5	24.4
38	7.3	13.2	23.9
39	7.2	12.7	22.6
40	7.1	12.3	21.4
41	7.0	11.6	19.4
42	6.9	11.0	17.5

An AFI below the 5th percentile is suggestive of oligohydramnios, and above the 95th percentile is suggestive of polyhydramnios. However, the validity of this table for diagnosis of oligohydramnios and polyhydramnios has not been clearly established. The ultrasound diagnosis of increased normal or decreased fluid should be complemented by the sonographer's subjective analysis.

FURTHER READING
Moore TR. Clinical assessment of amniotic fluid. *Clinical Obstetrics and Gynecology* 1997;**40**:303–313.

REFERENCE
1. Moore TR, Cayle JE. The amniotic fluid index in normal human pregnancy. *American Journal of Obstetrics and Gynecology* 1990;**162**:1168–1173.

INDEX

abdominal aorta 214–16
abdominal circumference (AC), fetal
    266–9, 270, 271–3
  birth weight estimation 276–85,
    318–19
  head circumference ratio 274–5
  thoracic circumference ratio 302
abdominal imaging
  common bile duct 14–19
  diaphragmatic motion 26–7
  gallbladder 6–11
  gallbladder wall 12–13
  hepatic duct 20–1
  liver 2–5
  pediatric
    common bile duct 18–19
    gallbladder 8–11
    liver 4–5
    spleen 23–5
  spleen 23–5
  vascular
    acute renal obstruction 34–5
    celiac artery 42–3, 46–7
    hepatic artery 40–1
    hepatic veins 38–9
    inferior mesenteric artery 48–50
    portal vein 36–7
    postprandial blood flow 46–7
    renal artery 30–2
    superior mesenteric artery 42,
      44, 46–7
  see also obstetric imaging
abductor pollicis longus 192, 193
acetabulum, developmental dysplasia
  of hip 198, 199
Achilles tendon 204–5
adenoma, parathyroid 134, 135
adrenal glands
  adult 66
  pediatric 67–9
amniotic fluid 320–2

amniotic fluid index (AFI) 320, 322
anal endosonography 170–1
anisotropic artifacts 175
ankle 202–3
antenatal imaging see obstetric
  imaging
anterior joint space of elbow 184–5
anterior tibial artery 218
  see also lower limb, arteries, stenosis
aorta
  abdominal 214–16
  pancreas transplants 92
  renal transplants 86
  renal–aortic ratio 30
appendicitis 164
appendix 164–5
appendix epididymis 108
appendix testis 104
arcuate arteries of kidney 34, 35
arteries, vein-to-artery ratio 240
  see also vascular system
artifacts, musculoskeletal imaging
  175
axillary artery 212

basilar artery 230, 232
biceps tendon 176–7
bile ducts
  adult 14–17, 20–1
  pediatric 18–19
biparietal diameter (BPD) 258–61,
  270, 271–3
  birth weight estimation 276–85,
    318–19
  and orbital diameters 308–11
bladder
  pancreas transplants 92
  residual volume 96–8
  ureterovesical jets 102–3
  volume 96–8
  wall 100–1

bowel
  endoscopic ultrasound 166
  fetal 312, 314–15, 316–17
  wall of 168–9
brachial artery 212
brachiocephalic (innominate) vein
  238
brain
  fetal
    cerebral ventricles 298–9
    cisterna magna 300–1
    intracranial blood flow 158–9,
      230–3
  neonatal
    intracranial blood flow 158–9
    ventricular size 154–7
bursae
  appearance 174
  interdigital 208
  retrocalcaneal 204
  suprapatellar 200

calcaneus 204, 205, 206, 207
carotid arteries 222–9, 230
carpal tunnel 194–5
carpal tunnel syndrome 194
cavernosal artery 114, 115
celiac artery (CA) 42–3, 46–7
  pancreas transplants 92
cerebral arteries 231, 232
  neonatal 158, 159
cerebral ventricles
  fetal 298–9
  neonates 154–7
  ventricular ratio (VR) 156
cerebrovascular disease, plaques 222
cervical canal 130–1
cervix 122–3
  in pregnancy 130–1
Chiari malformation 300
children see pediatric ultrasound
cholecystectomy, bile duct diameter
  after 14
cholecystitis, gallbladder wall
  thickness 12

chromosomal disorders
  cisterna magna 300
  nuchal fold thickness 254
  nuchal translucency thickness 256
cirrhosis
  hepatic veins 38
  portal vein, congestion index 36
cisterna magna, fetal 300–1
colon 168, 169
  fetal 314, 316–17
common bile duct
  adult 14–17
  pediatric 18–19
common carotid artery (CCA) 222,
  223
common iliac artery 214–16, 218
  pancreas transplants 92
common iliac vein, pancreas
  transplants 92
congestion index (CI), portal vein 36
crown–rump length, fetal 250, 251,
  252–3
cystic duct 18
cystic hygroma 256

developmental dysplasia of the hip
  198–9
diaphragmatic motion 26–7
Doppler perfusion index (DPI) 40
Doppler sonography
  acute renal obstruction 34–5
  appendix 164
  celiac artery 42–3, 46–7
  extracranial arteries 222, 223,
    226–9
  fetal heartbeat 250–1
  hepatic artery 40–1, 88, 89, 90
  hepatic veins 38–9, 88, 89, 90
  inferior mesenteric artery 48–50
  inferior vena cava 88, 90
  intracranial blood flow 158–9,
    230–3
  leg veins 240–2
  liver transplants 88–91
  lower limb arteries 218–19, 220–1

lymph nodes in neck 144, 145
neck veins 238–9
pancreas transplants 92–3
parathyroid adenoma 134
penile vascular system 114–16
portal vein 36–7, 88, 90, 91, 92
postprandial intestinal blood flow 46–7
renal artery 30–1, 86–7
renal transplants 82, 84, 86–7
superior mesenteric artery 42, 44, 46–7
thyroid arteries 142
umbilical arteries 294–7
upper limb arteries 212–13
ureterovesical jets 102–3
dorsal tendons, wrist 192–3
Down's syndrome
nuchal fold thickness 254
nuchal translucency thickness 256
duodenal atresia 312
duodenal walls 166

effusions, joint see synovial fluid
ejaculatory duct 112
elbow
anterior joint space 184–5
lateral 188–9
medial 190–1
olecranon fossa 186–7
elderly people
common bile duct 14, 16
kidney size 54
pancreas 70
end diastolic velocity (EDV)
basilar artery 232
cavernosal artery 114, 116
celiac artery 46–7
cerebral arteries 232
inferior mesenteric artery 48, 49
internal carotid artery 226, 228, 229
superior mesenteric artery 46–7
thyroid arteries 142
umbilical arteries 294

vertebral artery 232
end systolic velocity, neck veins 238
endometrial stripe 126–7
endoscopic ultrasound
anal canal 170–1
upper GI tract wall 166–7
epididymis 108–9
erectile dysfunction 114–16
extensor carpi radialis brevis 192, 193
extensor carpi radialis longus 192, 193
extensor carpi ulnaris 192
extensor digiti minimi 192
extensor digitorum 192, 193
extensor digitorum longus 202
extensor hallucis longus 202
extensor indicis 192, 193
extensor pollicis brevis 192, 193
extensor pollicis longus 192, 193
external anal sphincter (EAS) 170–1
external carotid artery (ECA) 222, 223, 224
external iliac artery, renal transplants 86
extracorporeal membrane oxygenation (ECMO) 158
extracranial arteries 222–9

female genital tract see genital tract, female
femoral artery 218, 219, 221
femoral vein 240, 241, 242
femur
fetal, length 270, 271–3, 286–9
hip imaging 197, 198, 199
knee imaging 200, 201
fetal imaging see obstetric imaging
fibular collateral ligament 200
flexor digitorum longus 202, 203
flexor digitorum profundus 194
flexor digitorum superficialis 194
flexor hallucis longus 202, 203
flexor retinaculum 194
food, postprandial blood flow 46–7

foot
  Achilles tendon insertion 204, 205
  interdigital web spaces 208–9
  plantar fascia 206–7

gallbladder
  adult 6–7
  pediatric 8–11
  wall thickness 12–13
gastric walls 166
gastrointestinal tract
  anal endosonography 170–1
  appendix 164–5
  bowel wall 168–9
  fetal colon 314, 316–17
  fetal small bowel 312, 314–15
  fetal stomach diameter 312–13
  postprandial intestinal blood flow
    46–7
  pyloric stenosis 162–3
  upper GI tract wall 166–7
genital tract
  female
    amniotic fluid volume 320–2
    cervix 122–3, 130–1
    endometrial stripe 126–7
    ovarian follicles 120–1
    ovary 118–19
    uterus 124–5, 126–7, 320–2
  male
    epididymis 108–9
    penis 114–16
    prostate 110–12
    seminal vesicles 112–13
    testes 104–6
gestational sac 244, 246–9
Graf alpha angle 198

head circumference, fetal 262–5,
  270, 271–3
  abdomen circumference ratio
    274–5
heartbeat, fetal 250–1
hepatic artery 40–1
  liver transplants 88, 89, 90

tardus parvus waveform 88, 89, 90
hepatic dimensions
  adult 2–3
  pediatric 4–5
hepatic duct, adult 20–1
hepatic transplantation 88–91
hepatic veins 38–9
  liver transplants 88, 89, 90
hip
  developmental dysplasia 198–9
  effusion 196–7
Hirschsprung's disease 316
β-human chorionic gonadotrophin
  (HCG) 244–5, 246
humerus
  capitellum 184, 185
  fetal, length 290–3
  lateral epicondyle of 188, 189
  medial epicondyle of 190, 191
hydrocephalus 158, 298
hydronephrosis
  fetal 304
  neonatal 64
hypertension, pregnancy-induced 294
hypoxic–ischemic brain injury 158

ileal atresia 314
iliac arteries 86, 92, 214–16, 218
iliac veins 92
iliacus muscle 76
iliotibial band 200
impotence, vasculogenic 114–16
infants
  adrenal glands 67–9
  brain 154–9
  common bile duct 18
  developmental dysplasia of hip
    198–9
  gallbladder 10–11
  kidneys 60–2, 64–5
  pancreas 74
  pyloric stenosis 162–3
  splenic length 22
  thyroid gland 140
  ureterovesical jets 102–3

inferior mesenteric artery 48–50
inferior vena cava (IVC) 236–7
   and hepatic veins 38, 39
      liver transplants 88, 89, 90
infraspinatus tendon 182–3
innominate (brachiocephalic) vein 238
interdigital web spaces 208–9
internal carotid artery (ICA) 222, 223, 224, 230
   neonates 158
   stenosis 226–9
internal jugular vein 238
intestinal tract *see* gastrointestinal tract
intimal-medial thickness (IMT), carotid artery 223, 225
intracranial anatomy, fetal 298–301
intracranial blood flow 230–3
   neonates 158–9

jejunal atresia 314
joint effusions *see* synovial fluid
jugular veins 238, 239

kidneys
   acute obstruction 34–5
   adult 52–4
   fetal 64–5, 304–5, 306–7
   neonatal 60–2, 64–5
   pediatric 56–65
   renal artery 30–2, 86–7
   transplantation 82–4, 86–7
knee 200–1

large bowel
   fetal 314, 316–17
   wall 168, 169
leg *see* lower limb
ligaments
   appearance 174
   elbow 188, 190
   knee 200
limbs *see* lower limb; upper limb
liver

adult 2–3
   cirrhosis 38
   hepatic artery 40–1, 88, 89, 90
   hepatic duct 20–1
   hepatic veins 38–9, 88, 89, 90
   inferior vena cava 88, 89, 90
   pediatric 4–5
   portal vein 36–7, 88, 90, 91
   transplantation 88–91
long head of biceps 176–7
lower limb
   Achilles tendon 204–5
   ankle 202–3
   arteries 218–19
      stenosis 220–1
   foot 206–9
   hip 196–9
   knee 200–1
   veins 240–2
lymph nodes
   cervical 144–6
   retroperitoneal 78–9

male genital tract *see* genital tract, male
malleolus 202, 203
meals, postprandial blood flow 46–7
mean sac diameter (MSD) 244, 246, 248
mean velocity (V_{mean}), inferior mesenteric artery 48
meconium ileus 314
median nerve 194, 195
mediastinum testis 104
metatarsals 208, 209
Morton's neuroma 208, 209
muscle bundles, appearance 174
musculoskeletal system 174–5
   artifacts 175
   bursae 174, 200, 204, 208
   ligaments 174, 188, 190, 200
   lower limb
      Achilles tendon 204–5
      ankle 202–3
      foot 206–9

musculoskeletal system cont.
  lower limb cont.
    hip 196–9
    knee 200–1
  muscle bundles 174
  nerves 174, 194, 195
  tendons
    artifacts 175
    general appearance 174
    see also specific tendons
  upper limb
    elbow 184–91
    shoulder 176–83
    wrist 192–5

neck veins 238–9
neonates
  adrenal glands 67, 68–9
  brain
    intracranial blood flow 158–9
    ventricular size 154–7
  common bile duct 18
  gallbladder 10–11
  kidneys 60–2, 64–5
  pancreas 74
  premature
    intracranial blood flow 158
    ventricular size 154, 156
  renal obstruction 64
  splenic length 22
  thyroid gland 140
nerves
  appearance 174
  carpal tunnel 194, 195
  optic nerve 150–1
neuromas, foot 208, 209
nuchal fold thickness 254–5
nuchal translucency (NT) thickness
  256–7

obstetric imaging
  amniotic fluid 320–2
  amniotic fluid index 320, 322
  birth weight estimation 276–84,
    318–19

cervix/cervical canal length 130–1
fetal abdominal circumference
  266–9, 270, 271–3
  birth weight estimation 276–85,
    318–19
  head circumference ratio 274–5
  thoracic circumference ratio
    302
fetal biparietal diameter 258–61,
  270, 271–3
  birth weight estimation 276–85,
    318–19
  and orbital diameters 308–11
fetal calvaria 258
fetal cerebral ventricles 298–9
fetal choroid plexi 298
fetal cisterna magna 300–1
fetal colon 314, 316–17
fetal crown–rump length 250, 251,
  252–3
fetal femur length 270, 271–3,
  286–9
fetal head circumference 262–5,
  270, 271–3, 274–5
fetal heartbeat 250–1
fetal humerus length 290–3
fetal orbital diameters 308–11
fetal renal length 306–7
fetal renal pelvis diameter 64–5,
  304–5
fetal small bowel 314–15
fetal stomach diameter 312–13
fetal thalami 258, 259
fetal thoracic circumference 302–3
fetal umbilical arteries 294–7
fetal weight percentiles 318–19
gestational age
  abdominal circumference 268–9,
    270, 271–3, 275
  amniotic fluid index 322
  biparietal diameter 260–1, 270,
    271–3
  birth weight prediction 318–19
  colon diameter 316
  crown–rump length 252–3

femur length 270, 271–3, 286–9
and gestational sac size 246,
    248
head circumference 264–5, 270,
    271–3, 275
β-hCG levels compared 244–5
humerus length 290–3
multiple fetal parameters 270–3
orbital diameters 308–11
renal length 306–7
small bowel diameter 314
stomach diameter 312–13
ultrasound landmarks compared
    244–5
umbilical artery 296
gestational sac 244, 246–9
β-hCG levels 244–5, 246
mean sac diameter 244, 246, 248
nuchal fold thickness 254–5
nuchal translucency thickness
    256–7
placental dysfunction 294
yolk sac 244, 246
oesophagus 166
older people see elderly people
olecranon fossa 186–7
oligohydramnios 322
ophthalmic artery 230
optic nerve 150–1
orbits
extraocular muscles 148–9
fetal, diameters 308–11
optic nerve 150–1
organ transplantation
kidney 82–4, 86–7
liver 88–91
pancreas 92–3
ovary 118–19
follicles 120–1

pancreas
adult 70–1, 72–3
pancreatic duct 72–3
pediatric 74–5
transplantation 92–3

pancreatitis 72
parathyroid glands 134–5
parotid salivary glands 138–9
patellar tendon 200, 201
peak systolic velocity (PSV)
basilar artery 232
cavernosal artery 114, 115, 116
celiac artery 42, 43, 46
cerebral arteries 232
inferior mesenteric artery 48, 49
internal carotid artery 226, 228,
    229
lower limb arteries 218, 220, 221
renal artery 30, 31, 86, 87
renal transplants 86, 87
superior mesenteric artery 42, 44,
    46
thyroid arteries 142
umbilical arteries 294
vertebral artery 232
pediatric ultrasound
adrenal glands 67–9
brain (neonatal) 154–9
common bile duct 18–19
developmental dysplasia of hip
    198–9
gallbladder 8–11
hip effusion 196–7
kidneys 56–62, 64–5
liver 4–5
ovary 118
pancreas 74–5
pyloric stenosis 162–3
renal obstruction 64
renal pelvis diameter 64–5
spleen 23–5
thyroid gland 140
ureterovesical jets 102–3
uterus 124
pelvis
bladder
    residual volume 96–8
    ureterovesical jets 102–3
    volume 96–8
    wall 100–1

pelvis cont.
  female urogenital tract
    cervix 122–3, 130–1
    endometrial stripe 126–7
    ovarian follicles 120–1
    ovary 118–21
    urethra 128–9
    uterus 124–7
  male genital tract
    epididymis 108–9
    penis 114–16
    prostate 110–12
    seminal vesicles 112–13
    testes 104–6
  pediatric, ureterovesical jets 102–3
penis 114–16
peripheral nerves
  appearance 174
  carpal tunnel 194, 195
peripheral vascular system *see*
  vascular system
peroneal artery 218
  see also lower limb, arteries,
    stenosis
peroneal tendons 202, 203
Peyronie's disease 114
pisiform 194, 195
placental dysfunction 294
plantar fascia, foot 206–7
plaques, extracranial arteries 222–4
polyhydramnios 322
popliteal artery 218
  see also lower limb, arteries,
    stenosis
popliteal vein 240
popliteus tendon 200
portal vein 36–7
  liver transplants 88, 90, 91
  pancreas transplants 92
posterior tibial artery 218
  see also lower limb, arteries,
    stenosis
postprandial intestinal blood flow
  46–7
pregnancy *see* obstetric imaging

pregnancy-induced hypertension 294
premature neonates
  intracranial blood flow 158
  ventricular size 154, 156
profunda femoris 218
prostate gland 110–12
psoas muscle 76–7
pulmonary hypoplasia 302
pulsatility index (PI) 46
  celiac artery 46
  inferior mesenteric artery 48
  superior mesenteric artery 46
pyloric stenosis 162–3

quadriceps tendon 200, 201

radial artery 212
radial head
  anterior joint space 184, 185
  lateral elbow 188, 189
recti muscles, extraocular 148–9
renal–aortic ratio (RAR) 30
renal arcuate arteries 34, 35
renal artery 30–2
  renal transplants 86–7
renal artery stenosis (RAS) 30, 31,
  32, 86–7
renal dimensions
  adult 52–4
  fetal 64–5, 304–5, 306–7
  neonatal 60–2, 64–5
  pediatric 56–65
renal obstruction
  acute 34–5
  neonates 64
renal transplantation 82–4
  renal artery stenosis in 86–7
residual volume, bladder 96–8
resistance index (RI) 30
  acute renal obstruction 34
  basilar artery 232
  cerebral arteries 232
    neonates 158, 159
  hepatic artery 40
    tardus parvus waveform 90

inferior mesenteric artery 48, 49
normal renal 30
pancreas transplants 92, 93
renal artery stenosis 30, 31, 32, 86
renal transplants 82, 84, 86
vertebral artery 232
rete testis 104
retroperitoneum
adrenal glands 66–9
kidneys 52–62, 64–5, 82–7
lymph nodes 78–9
pancreas 70–5
pancreatic duct 72–3
pediatric
adrenal glands 67–9
kidneys 56–62, 64–5
pancreas 74–5
renal pelvis diameter 64–5
psoas muscle 76–7

salivary glands
parotid 138–9
submandibular 136–7
scrotal ultrasound
epididymis 108–9
testes 104–6
secretin administration, pancreatic
duct 72
seminal vesicles 112–13
shoulder
infraspinatus tendon 182–3
long head of biceps 176–7
subscapularis tendon 178–9
supraspinatus tendon 180–1
teres minor tendon 182
small bowel
endoscopic ultrasound 166
fetal 312, 314–15
wall thickness 168
spleen 23–5
stomach
endoscopic ultrasound 166–7
fetal, diameter 312–13
wall thickness 168
'string-flow' 226

subclavian artery 212, 213
subclavian vein 238
submandibular salivary glands
136–7
subscapularis tendon 178–9
superficial structures
cervical lymph nodes 144–6
orbits
extraocular muscles 148–9
optic nerve 150–1
parathyroid glands 134–5
parotid salivary glands 138–9
submandibular salivary glands
136–7
thyroid gland 140–2
superficial veins 240, 241, 242
superior mesenteric artery (SMA) 42,
44, 46–7, 92
suprapatellar pouch 200, 201
supraspinatus tendon 180–1
synovial fluid
ankle 202
elbow 184, 185
hindfoot 204
hip 196–7
systolic/diastolic (S/D) ratio,
umbilical arteries 294–7
see also end diastolic velocity; peak
systolic velocity

tardus parvus waveform 88, 89, 90
tendons
artifacts 175
general appearance 174
see also specific tendons
teres minor tendon 182
testes 104–6
epididymis 108–9
thoracic circumference, fetal 302–3
thrombosis
hepatic artery 88
inferior vena cava 90
leg veins 240–2
portal vein 88
thyroid arteries 142

thyroid gland 140–2
  and parathyroid 134, 135
thyroid veins 142
tibia, knee imaging 200, 201
tibialis anterior 202
tibialis posterior tendon 202, 203
tibiotalar joint 202
transcranial Doppler ultrasound
    158–9, 230–3
transorbital Doppler ultrasound 230
transplantation
  kidney 82–4, 86–7
  liver 88–91
  pancreas 92–3
transrectal sonography
  prostate 110–12
  seminal vesicles 112–13
transvaginal sonography (TVS)
  cervix 122–3, 130
  obstetrics
    crown–rump length 252
    fetal heartbeat 250
    gestational sac 244, 246–7
    nuchal translucency thickness
      256
    and serum β-hCG levels 244–5,
      246
  ovary 118–19
    follicles 120–1
  uterus 124–5
    endometrial stripe 126–7
trisomy 21 syndrome see Down's
    syndrome

ulnar artery 212
ulnar collateral ligaments 188, 190
umbilical arteries 294–7
upper limb
  arteries 212–13
  elbow
    anterior joint space 184–5
    lateral 188–9
    medial 190–1
    olecranon fossa 186–7
  shoulder

infraspinatus tendon 182–3
long head of biceps 176–7
subscapularis tendon 178–9
supraspinatus tendon 180–1
wrist
  carpal tunnel 194–5
  dorsal tendons 192–3
ureterovesical jets 102–3
urethra, female 128–9
urinary tract
  bladder
    residual volume 96–8
    ureterovesical jets 102–3
    volume 96–8
    wall 100–1
  fetal 304
  kidneys see kidneys
  urethra, female 128–9
uterus 124–5
  amniotic fluid volume 320–2
  endometrial stripe 126–7

varicocele 106
vascular system
  abdominal aorta 214–16
  acute renal obstruction 34–5
  celiac artery 42–3, 46–7
  common iliac artery 214–16
  extracranial arteries 222–9
  hepatic artery 40–1, 88, 89, 90
  hepatic veins 38–9, 88, 89, 90
  inferior mesenteric artery 48–50
  inferior vena cava 236–7
    and hepatic veins 38, 39, 88, 89,
      90
    liver transplants 88, 89, 90
  internal carotid artery stenosis
      226–9
  intracranial blood flow 230–3
    neonates 158–9
  liver transplants 88–91
  lower limb arteries 218–21
  lower limb veins 240–2
  neck veins 238–9
  pancreas transplants 92–3

penile 114–16
portal vein 36–7, 88, 90, 91, 92
postprandial blood flow 46–7
renal artery 30–2, 86–7
renal transplants 82, 84, 86–7
superior mesenteric artery 42, 44,
    46–7
thyroid arteries 142
thyroid veins 142
transcranial Doppler 158–9,
    230–3
umbilical arteries 294–7
upper limb arteries 212–13
vein-to-artery ratio 240

veins *see* vascular system
ventricles, cerebral
    fetal 298–9
    neonates 154–7
ventricular ratio (VR) 156
vertebral artery (VA) 222, 223, 230,
    232
volvulus 314, 316

wrist
    carpal tunnel 194–5
    dorsal tendons 192–3

yolk sac 244, 246